Diseases of
the Mediastinum

Guest Editor

FEDERICO VENUTA, MD

THORACIC
SURGERY CLINICS

www.thoracic.theclinics.com

Consulting Editor
MARK K. FERGUSON, MD

February 2009 • Volume 19 • Number 1

SAUNDERS an imprint of ELSEVIER, Inc.

W.B. SAUNDERS COMPANY
A Division of Elsevier Inc.

1600 John F. Kennedy Boulevard • Suite 1800 • Philadelphia, Pennsylvania 19103-2899

http://www.theclinics.com

THORACIC SURGERY CLINICS Volume 19, Number 1
February 2009 ISSN 1547-4127, ISBN-13: 978-1-4377-0551-5, ISBN-10: 1-4377-0551-0

Editor: Catherine Bewick
Developmental Editor: Theresa Collier

Thoracic Surgery Clinics (ISSN 1547-4127) is published quarterly by Elsevier Inc., 360 Park Avenue South, New York, NY 10010-1710. Months of publication are February, May, August, and November. Business and editorial offices: 1600 John F. Kennedy Boulevard, Suite 1800, Philadelphia, PA 19103-2899. Customer service office: 11830 Westline Industrial Drive, St. Louis, MO 63146. Periodicals postage paid at New York, NY, and additional mailing offices. Subscription prices are $242.00 per year (US individuals), $360.00 per year (US institutions), $121.00 per year (US students), $309.00 per year (Canadian individuals), $455.00 per year (Canadian institutions), $165.00 per year (Canadian and foreign students), $329.00 per year (foreign individuals), and $455.00 per year (foreign institutions). Foreign air speed delivery is included in all *Clinics'* subscription prices. All prices are subject to change without notice. **POSTMASTER:** Send address changes to *Thoracic Surgery Clinics,* Elsevier Journals Customer Service, 11830 Westline Industrial Drive, St. Louis, MO 63146. **Customer Service: 1-800-654-2452 (US and Canada). From outside of the US and Canada, call 1-314-453-7041. Fax: 1-314-453-5170. For print support, e-mail: JournalsCustomerService-usa@elsevier.com. For online support, e-mail: JournalsOnlineSupport-usa@elsevier.com.**

Reprints. For copies of 100 or more, of articles in this publication, please contact Commercial Rights Department, Elsevier Inc., 360 Park Avenue South, New York, NY 10010-1710. Tel: (212) 633-3812; Fax: (212) 462-1935; E-mail: reprints@elsevier.com.

Thoracic Surgery Clinics is covered in *MEDLINE/PubMed (Index Medicus)* and *EMBASE/Excerpta Medica.*

Printed and bound by CPI Group (UK) Ltd, Croydon, CR0 4YY

Transferred to Digital Print 2012

Contributors

CONSULTING EDITOR

MARK K. FERGUSON, MD
Professor of Surgery, Section of Cardiac and
Thoracic Surgery, The University of Chicago,
Chicago, Illinois

GUEST EDITOR

FEDERICO VENUTA, MD
Associate Professor of Thoracic Surgery,
Head Lung Transplantation Program, Department
of Thoracic Surgery, Policlinico Umberto I,
University "La Sapienza" of Rome, Rome, Italy

AUTHORS

CLEMENS AIGNER, MD
Medical University of Vienna, Vienna, Austria

KALLIOPIA A. ATHANASSIADI, MD, PhD
Consultant Cardiothoracic Surgeon,
Department of Thoracic Surgery, General
Hospital of Piraeus, Athens, Greece

WAQAS ANJUM, MD
Department of Cardiothoracic Surgery, Drexel
University College of Medicine, Philadelphia,
Pennsylvania

PERCY BOATENG, MD
Assistant Professor, Department of
Cardiothoracic Surgery, Drexel University
College of Medicine, Philadelphia,
Pennsylvania

KEVIN S. CHOE, MD
Department of Radiation and Cellular
Oncology, University of Chicago, Chicago,
Illinois

GIORGIO F. COLONI, MD
Professor of Thoracic Surgery and Head,
Thoracic Surgery Unit, Department of Surgery,
University of Rome Sapienza, Policlinico
Umberto I, Rome, Italy

JOEL D. COOPER, MD
Professor of Surgery and Chief, Division
of Thoracic Surgery, Hospital of the University
of Pennsylvania, Philadelphia, Pennsylvania

HIROSHI DATE, MD
Professor and Chairman, Department
of Thoracic Surgery, Kyoto University,
Graduate School of Medicine, Kyoto, Japan

PIA DI BENEDETTO, MD
Department of Anesthesiology, University
of Rome "La Sapienza," Ospedale S. Andrea,
Rome, Italy

LAWRENCE H. EINHORN, MD
Professor of Medicine, Department of
Medicine, Hematology/Oncology Division,
Indiana University School of Medicine,
Indianapolis, Indiana

PIER LUIGI FILOSSO, MD
Assistant Professor of Thoracic Surgery,
Division of Thoracic Surgery, University of
Torino, Torino, Italy

MIR ALI REZA HODA, MD
Medical University of Vienna, Vienna, Austria

DAVID R. JONES, MD
Professor of Surgery and Chief, Division of
Thoracic and Cardiovascular Surgery; and
Chief, General Thoracic Surgery, Department
of Surgery, University of Virginia,
Charlottesville, Virginia

KENNETH A. KESLER, MD
Professor of Surgery, Department of Surgery,
Cardiothoracic Division, Indiana University
School of Medicine, Indianapolis, Indiana

WALTER KLEPETKO, MD
Professor of Thoracic Surgery, Medical
University of Vienna, Vienna, Austria

JOHN C. KUCHARCZUK, MD
Assistant Professor of Surgery, Division
of Thoracic Surgery, Hospital of the University
of Pennsylvania, Philadelphia, Pennsylvania

MICHAEL J. MACK, MD
Chairman of the Board, Cardiopulmonary
Research Science Technology Institute, Dallas;
and Medical Director, The Heart Hospital at
Baylor Plano, Plano, Texas

MITCHELL J. MAGEE, MD
Director, Minimally Invasive Thoracic Surgery
and Surgical Oncology; and Chief,
Cardiothoracic Surgery, Medical City Dallas
Hospital, Cardiopulmonary Research Science
Technology Institute, Dallas, Texas

DOMENICO MASSULLO, MD
Department of Anesthesiology, University
of Rome "La Sapienza," Ospedale S. Andrea,
Rome, Italy

BRYAN F. MEYERS, MD, MPH
Division of Cardiothoracic Surgery,
Washington University School of Medicine,
Barnes-Jewish Hospital, St. Louis, Missouri

ALBERTO OLIARO, MD
Professor of Thoracic Surgery, Division of
Thoracic Surgery, University of Torino, Torino,
Italy

GIOVANNI PINTO, MD
Professor of Anesthesiology and Head,
Department of Anesthesiology, University
of Rome "La Sapienza," Ospedale S. Andrea,
Rome, Italy

VARUN PURI, MD
Division of Cardiothoracic Surgery,
Washington University School of Medicine,
Barnes-Jewish Hospital, St. Louis,
Missouri

PHILIP A. RASCOE, MD
Instructor, Division of Thoracic Surgery,
Hospital of the University of Pennsylvania,
Philadelphia, Pennsylvania

ERINO A. RENDINA, MD
Professor of Thoracic Surgery and Head,
Thoracic Surgery Unit, University of Rome
Sapienza, Ospedale S. Andrea, Rome,
Italy

ENRICO RUFFINI, MD
Associate Professor of Thoracic Surgery,
Division of Thoracic Surgery, University
of Torino, Torino, Italy

JOSEPH K. SALAMA, MD
Department of Radiation and Cellular
Oncology; Cancer Research Center; and
Ludwig Center for Metastases Research,
University of Chicago, Chicago, Illinois

MATTHEW D. TAYLOR, MD
Post-Doctorate Fellow and Resident,
Department of Surgery, University of Virginia,
Charlottesville, Virginia

FEDERICO VENUTA, MD
Associate Professor of Thoracic Surgery,
Head Lung Transplantation Program, Department
of Thoracic Surgery, Policlinico Umberto I,
University "La Sapienza" of Rome, Rome, Italy

ANDREW S. WECHSLER, MD
Professor and Chair, Department of
Cardiothoracic Surgery, Drexel University
College of Medicine, Philadelphia,
Pennsylvania

CAMERON D. WRIGHT, MD
Section Chief, Division of Thoracic Surgery,
Massachusetts General Hospital; and
Associate Professor of Surgery,
Harvard Medical School, Boston,
Massachusetts

Contents

Surgery of the Mediastinum: Historical Notes   1

Philip A. Rascoe, John C. Kucharczuk, and Joel D. Cooper

> Surgical management of diseases of the mediastinum ushered in the era of chest surgery, as the risks of exploration of the pleural spaces were prohibitive until the advent of positive-pressure ventilation. Early procedures were undertaken for suppurative and tuberculous bacterial infections. These approaches were subsequently applied for extirpation of primary and secondary neoplasms of the mediastinum. Finally, less invasive techniques for the diagnosis of mediastinal processes and the staging of bronchogenic carcinoma were developed. This article discusses the historical perspectives of mediastinal surgery.

Utility of Positron Emission Tomography in the Mediastinum: Moving Beyond Lung and Esophageal Cancer Staging   7

Varun Puri and Bryan F. Meyers

> Functional imaging using positron emission tomography (PET) has been a major advance in tumor imaging over the last decade. Its role is established in breast cancer, colorectal cancer, nonsmall cell lung cancer, and lymphoma. This article discusses the indications and applications of PET to evaluate mediastinal pathology.

Genetic Markers of Mediastinal Tumors   17

Matthew D. Taylor and David R. Jones

> Most adult mediastinal tumors are thymic in nature, and only more recently has there been scientific inquiry into the molecular biology and genetic alterations associated with these tumors. There is an increasing appreciation of specific genetic polymorphisms in myasthenia gravis and associated thymoma. In addition, thymic tumor progression is regulated by perturbations in expression of specific tumor suppressor genes and signal transduction pathways important in oncogenesis. This article highlights the known genetic and signaling pathway alterations important in the tumor biology of mediastinal tumors, with emphasis on thymic tumors. It also discusses the association of genetic markers with thymoma, thymic carcinoma, germ cell tumors, lymphoma, and neurogenic tumors. New gene-based techniques have enabled scientists to uncover differential gene expression patterns between subtypes of thymomas, correlate tumor marker expression with germ cell tumors, and determine a link between the NF-κB and JAK/STAT pathways with Hodgkin's and non-Hodgkin's lymphoma. Additionally, the use of genetic analysis has uncovered an important role for various tumor suppressor genes in the pathogenesis of paraganglioma and pheochromocytoma.

> Many histologically different tumors and cysts that affect people of all ages arise from the multiple anatomic structures present in the mediastinum. The number of diagnostic possibilities can be narrowed by considering the patient's age, tumor location, the presence or absence of symptoms and signs, the association of a specific systemic disease, radiographic findings, and biochemical markers. Pathologic diagnosis is often required to confirm a presumed diagnosis and to select the optimal treatment modality. A variety of biopsy techniques for obtaining tissue from the mediastinum have been described, including ultrasound-guided endoscopic biopsy, percutaneous image-guided needle biopsy, parasternal anterior mediastinotomy, cervical mediastinoscopy, and video-assisted thoracoscopic surgery. The choice of biopsy technique depends on the localization of the lesion, clinical factors such as the age and the condition of the patient, and the availability of special techniques with the required expert and the equipment.

> Infections of the mediastinum (ie, mediastinitis) are serious, are associated with high morbidity and mortality, and may result from adjacent disease with direct extension, hematogenous spread, or direct introduction into the mediastinal space. The organs and tissues involved determine the manifestations and approach to treatment of these infections. The most common ones are those secondary to perforation of the esophagus or penetrating trauma, and those that extend from an adjacent infection. Today, the most common cause of mediastinitis is direct invasion of the mediastinum after surgical intervention. Cases of mediastinitis can be classified as either acute or chronic. Two broad categories of acute mediastinitis are acute necrotizing mediastinitis and poststernotomy mediastinitis. Chronic mediastinitis has been arbitrarily subdivided into two categories: (1) granulomatous mediastinitis, and (2) fibrosing or sclerosing mediastinitis. However, these likely represent a continuum of chronic infection. In cases of acute mediastinitis, treatment should always be directed toward the primary pathology and the clinical presentation. In chronic cases, surgical treatment is only palliative.

> Pediatric mediastinal tumors and cysts are rare disorders that share many similarities with adults, yet which have important differences unique to the child. Posterior mediastinal tumors are relatively more common in children than in adults and are also more likely to be malignant in children. CT imaging facilitates the diagnostic evaluation of mediastinal masses in children. Airway compression is always a concern with large mediastinal tumors in children given their relative softer and smaller airway.

> Germ cell tumors originating in the anterior mediastinal compartment represent a rare but biologically interesting group of neoplasms. Knowledge of the specific biologic behaviors and therapeutic strategies for the three histologic types is important. This article discusses the multimodality treatment strategy for primary mediastinal nonseminomatous germ cell tumors.

Multimodality Treatment of Thymic Tumors   71

Federico Venuta, Erino A. Rendina, and Giorgio F. Coloni

Tumors of the thymus are rather infrequent compared with all the other thoracic neo-plasms. They may display a variable clinical presentation and outcome. Although they may present as a capsulated lesion with an indolent course, in other cases they may be locally aggressive, invading the surrounding structures, or show the presence of distant metastases. At these advanced stages, cure and complete resection may be difficult, and only a multimodality approach integrating surgery with induction chemotherapy and adjuvant treatment can contribute to improve outcome.

Surgical Approaches to the Thymus in Patients with Myasthenia Gravis   83

Mitchell J. Magee and Michael J. Mack

Myasthenia gravis is an autoimmune disorder of neuromuscular transmission affect-ing 2 out of every 100,000 people. Neurologists and surgeons still debate what role surgery should play in its management. Many patients who might benefit from thy-mectomy are denied the opportunity because of misconceptions, ignorance, or trep-idation. By offering effective methods of less invasive thymectomy to these patients, a significant number of patients and treating neurologists previously unwilling to consider surgery may realize the benefits of this established, proven treatment alter-native. The surgical approaches reviewed include: transcervical, videothoraco-scopic, robotic-assisted, transsternal, and combined transcervical–transsternal maximal thymectomy.

Vascular Lesions of the Mediastinum   91

Percy Boateng, Waqas Anjum, and Andrew S. Wechsler

This article highlights the vascular lesions that present as mediastinal masses. Some radiographic findings represent interesting clinical findings that do not require further intervention, such as a persistent left superior vena cava. Differentiating these find-ings from true pathologic entities then becomes paramount. In other cases, the clin-ical presentation will prompt immediate surgical or medical management to mitigate or prevent the mortality and morbidity associated with the condition, such as acute aortic dissection. Although specific details about the management of each clinical or pathologic entity are beyond the scope of this article, a brief mention is made of currently recommended therapy where appropriate.

Combined Cervicothoracic Approaches for Complex Mediastinal Masses   107

Clemens Aigner, Mir Ali Reza Hoda, and Walter Klepetko

The cervicothoracic junction is an anatomical complex region that contains impor-tant neurovascular structures as well as the central routes of the airway and upper digestive tract. Masses arising in either compartment—the mediastinum or the cer-vical region—may extensively involve the other one, requiring a combined surgical approach to achieve complete resection. The choice of the most appropriate ap-proach is therefore crucial and requires careful preoperative planning.

Intraoperative Strategy in Patients with Extended Involvement of Mediastinal Structures   113

Domenico Massullo, Pia Di Benedetto, and Giovanni Pinto

The mediastinum is a virtual space containing several vital organs and structures. Biopsy and resection of lesions located within this region often require several considerations that bear on intraoperative strategy. To optimize outcome, clinicians must be able to predict which patients are at highest risk of anesthetic complications. Superior vena cava involvement, extensive compression of the airway, and pericardial effusion have a clear impact on the decision-making of the anesthetist and surgeon, who should plan together when forming the surgical strategy.

Mediastinal neoplasms include various malignancies arising from structures anatomically located in this area and from adjacent organs. Treatment options in mediastinal tumors are chemotherapy, radiotherapy and surgery, or a combination of both. Although the role of surgery in the treatment of most mediastinal malignancies is well-established either alone or as part of a combined modality treatment, far less clear is the value of surgical resection for recurrent or chemorefractory mediastinal tumors. In particular, recurrent thymoma may take advantage from surgery that often allows complete resection and long-term survival.

Various malignancies either arise from or spread into the mediastinum. Radiotherapy in the area of the mediastinum is challenging because of the proximity to other critical organs, such as the heart, lungs, esophagus, and spinal cord. With recent advances in imaging, treatment, and the understanding of tumor biology, these diseases now can be treated more effectively and safely. This article reviews such innovations in radiotherapy and discusses their applications in tumors that involve the mediastinum.

Thoracic Surgery Clinics

THE CLINICS ARE NOW AVAILABLE ONLINE!

Access your subscription at:
www.theclinics.com

Preface

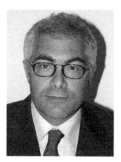

Federico Venuta, MD
Guest Editor

This issue of *Thoracic Surgery Clinics* focuses on the diseases of the mediastinum. This thoracic compartment is a sort of Pandora's box, able to give rise to a great number of fascinating clinical situations. Virtually any disorder originating within the neck or the chest can involve the mediastinum, as well as many systemic disorders; a multidisciplinary approach is often required for diagnosis, involving radiologists, internists, gastroenterologists, pulmonologists, neurologists, pediatricians, surgeons, and pathologists. In addition, treatment is usually designed by the medical and radiation oncologist and by the thoracic surgeon together, but in specific subsets, other experts may be required.

This contribution on mediastinal disorders has been designed to update the readers on many different aspects that involve the modern thoracic surgeon when dealing with this compartment: from diagnostic strategies with positron emission tomography, genetic markers, and surgical approaches, to the management of difficult situations with primary or recurring invasive tumors that require a multimodality approach. Other challenging topics, such as vascular lesions, extended resections, infections, and newly developed radiation strategies have been included.

All of the authors have been selected for their expertise and proven achievement in these challenging fields; I would like to sincerely thank all of them for participating with enthusiasm in this project. I hope that the different contributions will help the readers to fill in the gaps and stimulate them for future developments.

Federico Venuta, MD
Policlinico Umberto I
University "La Sapienza" of Rome
V.le del Policlinico155
00100 Rome
Italy

E-mail address:
federico.venuta@uniroma1.it

Thorac Surg Clin 19 (2009) xi
doi:10.1016/j.thorsurg.2008.11.001

Surgery of the Mediastinum: Historical Notes

Philip A. Rascoe, MD, John C. Kucharczuk, MD,
Joel D. Cooper, MD*

KEYWORDS

- Mediastinum • Thymectomy • Mediastinoscopy
- Mediastinitis

Mediastinal surgery, not unlike the entire field of thoracic surgery, has evolved in response to the maladies of the age. Mediastinal infections secondary to pyogenic and tuberculous organisms were drained by an extrapleural approach before the use of intratracheal positive-pressure anesthesia. As chest roentography became commonplace, tumors of the thorax were diagnosed more frequently. Before the 1920s, these were usually mediastinal in origin, as bronchogenic carcinoma was as yet exceedingly rare. Most mediastinal masses were initially irradiated, as physicians of the day were loath to refer patients for thoracic surgery. As median sternotomy and thoracotomy were proven to be safe, surgical series of resected mediastinal tumors proved that the majority of these tumors were benign, and thus curable with surgical resection. The demonstration that myasthenia gravis was often associated with abnormalities of the thymus gland led to increased performance of thymectomy for both tumors and hyperplasia. As the incidence of primary lung cancer rapidly increased, new procedures appeared to accurately sample and stage the mediastinal lymph nodes.

MILTON AND MEDIAN STERNOTOMY

Before 1897, only two operations for mediastinal disease had been recorded. The first, performed in 1872 at the Saint Louis Hospital in Paris, consisted of resection of a portion of the sternum and division of the remainder to resect a mediastinal growth. The second, performed by Bastinelli in 1893, consisted of a partial manubrectomy and resection of an anterior mediastinal dermoid cyst.[1]

As median sternotomy is the most common approach for cardiac surgery, it is often assumed that it was conceived as such. Rather, sternotomy was devised as an approach to the anterior mediastinum and predates cardiac surgery by five decades. The first modern median sternotomy was described by Herbert Milton, principal medical officer at the Kasr El Aini Hospital in Cairo, in 1897.[2] Before its clinical application, Milton performed and perfected median sternotomy in human cadavers at necropsy. He subsequently used this approach to explore the mediastinum of a live goat. Despite entry into both pleural spaces, he was able to continue the operation by performing immediate tracheostomy and providing ventilation with a glass tube and bellows. Following closure of the plurae and sternum and removal of the tracheostomy, the animal was ambulatory within half an hour.[3,4] Encouraged by this work, Milton used his approach in the treatment of a 25-year-old Egyptian farmer with infiltrating tuberculosis of the sternum and mediastinal lymph nodes. With the patient under chloroform anesthesia, Milton performed a median sternotomy, removed multiple caseous mediastinal nodes, and resected most of the sternum. The wound was packed with gauze and ultimately healed with frequent dressing changes. Summarizing his efforts, Milton concluded that, "undoubtedly the splitting of the

Division of Thoracic Surgery, Hospital of the University of Pennsylvania, 3400 Spruce Street, 6 Silverstein Pavilion, Philadelphia, PA 19104, USA
* Corresponding author.
E-mail address: joel.cooper@uphs.upenn.edu (J.D. Cooper).

Thorac Surg Clin 19 (2009) 1–5
doi:10.1016/j.thorsurg.2008.09.007

thoracic.theclinics.com

sternum affords the most perfect approach to the anterior and middle mediastina." "Milton's operation" was subsequently advocated as the approach to the anterior mediastinum in many of the early thoracic surgery texts.[2]

SUPPURATIVE MEDIASTINITIS

It had long been recognized that mediastinitis and pyogenic abscesses may result from contiguous pleural or pulmonary, ascending retroperitoneal, and descending cervical infectious processes. While the anatomic relationships of the neck and mediastinum had been previously described, Herman Pearse's publication regarding cervico-mediastinal fascial continuity and the surgical prevention and management of mediastinitis following cervical suppuration was indeed landmark.[5] In this article, Pearse noted that approximately 20% of cases of suppurative mediastinitis resulted from descending cervical infections, the majority as a result of cervical esophageal perforation. He identified the retrovisceral space as the most common path of dependent spread, and advocated early operative drainage via cervical mediastinotomy in such cases, noting 35% mortality in patients operated upon as compared with 85% mortality in the nonoperative group. For chronic mediastinal infections and those occurring below the sixth thoracic vertebra, he advocated drainage via posterior mediastinotomy. This approach to the mediastinum had been previously described by Howard Lilienthal[6] for an extrapleural resection of the esophagus for cancer.

MEDIASTINAL TUMORS

As tracheal intubation and administration of inhalational anesthetic agents under positive pressure became commonplace, operations for thoracic disease became less daunting. Moreover, routine performance of chest radiography led to the diagnosis of intrathoracic tumors more frequently. In the early to mid-nineteenth century, several surgical series of mediastinal tumors began to appear in the literature. In 1932, Harrington[7] reported on his experience with 23 cases of mediastinal tumors, noting that a large percentage of the tumors were benign and thus eminently curable with surgical resection alone. He also concluded that of the five tumors that were malignant and thus unresectable, three had probably undergone malignant degeneration. He therefore advocated resection of all benign asymptomatic mediastinal tumors, as they all have malignant potential. He further advocated exploratory thoracotomy for tumors in which the diagnosis was in question. However, for undiagnosed tumors that exhibited characteristics of primary lymphatic malignancy, he advocated a trial course of radiation therapy. Tumor response to radiation was virtually diagnostic of lymphatic malignancy, indicating that the patient should receive further radiation therapy rather than surgery. The majority of his resections were performed via a posterolateral transpleural approach.

Heuer[8] subsequently reported on his experience with 145 mediastinal tumors. Dermoid cysts and teratomas were the most frequently encountered tumors in his series. He commented that the majority of patients referred for surgical therapy had already received radiation therapy for their lesions, reflecting a prevalent opinion that all mediastinal tumors were radiosensitive and should be treated as such. Heuer suggested the reversal of this attitude, advocating consultation with a thoracic surgeon for all mediastinal tumors before initiating roentgenotherapy. He used an anterior T-shaped thoracotomy for tumors of the anterior mediastinum and posterolateral thoracotomy for those of the posterior mediastinum. It is interesting that neither Harrington nor Heuer mention median sternotomy in their series.

Blades[9] reported on 109 patients in the United States Army who underwent resection or attempted resection of a mediastinal tumor. In this series, neurogenic tumors, followed closely by bronchogenic cysts, were the most numerous. Like Heuer, Blades commented that the reticence of physicians to recommend exploratory thoracotomy led to the injudicious use of radiation therapy in many instances. He reported that in 114 exploratory operations, there were no deaths or postoperative complications when thoracotomy and biopsy alone were performed. This demonstrated the safety of exploration and attempted resection before institution of radiation therapy for tumors in which the diagnosis was in question.

Subsequently, Sabiston and Scott[10] published a series of 101 patients with tumors or cysts of the mediastinum treated at Johns Hopkins Hospital. Because of a preponderance of anterior mediastinal lesions, anterolateral thoracotomy was used most commonly. Median sternotomy was employed for superior mediastinal lesions, while neurogenic tumors and other posterior lesions were approached by posterolateral thoracotomy.

MYASTHENIA GRAVIS AND THYMECTOMY

The first report of a thymic tumor in association with myasthenia gravis was made by Weigert in 1901. In 1917, Bell reported on the autopsy findings of 57 patients who died of myasthenia gravis, finding thymic abnormalities in 27. Norris brought this series up to date in 1936, describing 35 thymic abnormalities in 80 necropsy cases.[11,12]

Thymectomy via neck incision was originally described in 1910 by Veau and Olivier as a proposed means to relieve upper airway obstruction in infants and children thought to be suffering from an enlarged thymus.[13] Von Haberer reported on 40 transcervical thymectomies performed for thyrotoxicosis, including one patient who also suffered from myasthenia gravis, in 1917.[11] Before 1939, the literature contained only four reports of attempts to influence the course of myasthenia gravis through surgical intervention. Three of these operations were performed by Sauerbruch and the fourth by Haberer. All were performed through the neck, with two patients reporting improvement in symptoms, and two dying of postoperative infection.[12]

In 1936, Alfred Blalock[12] removed a benign thymoma from a 19-year-old female patient with severe relapsing myasthenia gravis. He performed his operation via partial median sternotomy through the right third intercostal space. She had a smooth postoperative course and was discharged from the hospital 3 weeks later. Her symptoms and exercise tolerance improved considerably and she was eventually weaned from all medications. In his publication of this case report, Blalock commented, "If it is decided in the future that surgical exploration of the thymic region is indicated in patients with this disease, it should be performed through an approach which gives adequate exposure, such as division of the upper part of the sternum. One should not rely upon the imperfect view which is obtained through an incision in the lower part of the neck." Blalock subsequently reported on 20 patients who underwent thymectomy for myasthenia gravis, and Keynes reported on 260 such cases.[14,15] Their work led to the adoption of median sternotomy as the preferred approach for thymectomy, and transcervical thymectomy became something of a lost art.

Transcervical thymectomy was reintroduced by Crile in 1964[16] and subsequent reports by Carlens[17] and Kirschner[18] advocated its use in patients with myasthenia gravis. In 1988, Cooper and colleagues[19] reported modifications of the transcervical approach, which resulted in improved exposure and therefore greater assurance of complete thymectomy. Minimally invasive techniques using video-assisted thoracic surgery have since been introduced. There is still considerable debate regarding the optimal surgical approach for thymectomy in patients with myasthenia gravis in the absence of thymoma. Modern series of transcervical thymectomy in myasthenia patients report improvement in symptoms in at least 80% of patients, with 35% to 45% of them achieving complete remission.[20,21]

DIAGNOSTIC AND STAGING PROCEDURES

As diseases of the thorax became more readily treatable, advanced procedures were developed to obtain tissue for diagnosis. In 1949, Daniels[22] described the use of a supraclavicular incision to biopsy the ipsilateral scalene and upper mediastinal lymph nodes of patients with pulmonary conditions that were refractory to diagnosis by less invasive means. He reported five cases in which a diagnosis (three benign, two malignant) was obtained by this procedure, thus making exploratory thoracotomy unnecessary.

This procedure was expanded upon by Harken and colleagues.[23] Using the same inicision, they bluntly dissected through the cervical fascia into the superior mediastinum, sweeping the mediastinal pleura laterally so that the paratracheal lymph nodes could be exposed. Enlarged nodes were digitally enucleated, while fixed nodes were biopsied using a laryngoscope and laryngeal biopsy forceps. Based on Rouviere's initial description of lymphatic drainage of the lung,[24] they performed right cervicomediastinal exploration for right-sided pulmonary lesions, left cervicomediastinal exploration for left upper lobe lesions, and bilateral exploration for left lower lobe lesions. Overall, a positive histologic diagnosis was obtained in 32% of their patients. Moreover, in 40% of their patients ultimately proven to have bronchogenic carcinoma, they identified metastases to cervical or mediastinal lymph nodes that were not evident on physical examination. They noted that half of the positive results came from mediastinal nodes, and thus concluded that scalene fatpad excision alone was an inadequate diagnostic procedure. Based on these results, they advocated routine performance of this procedure in the evaluation of all patients with known or suspected bronchogenic carcinoma before thoracotomy. Patients with involved cervical or mediastinal nodes were deemed inoperable. In summarizing the value of this staging procedure, they stated " a technique that spares needless suffering for the hopelessly involved patient is as important as the extension of excisional therapy in an attempt to cure more people."

Most likely because of fear of complications (pneumothorax and injury to subclavian and jugular veins were described), the cervicomediastinal exploration described by Harken and colleagues was not widely adopted. Carlens[25] subsequently described a superior diagnostic procedure, cervical mediastinoscopy. This procedure was performed through an incision in the suprasternal notch and used blunt finger dissection to free the paratracheal nodes. Using a specially designed mediastinoscope, a blunt-tipped aspirator, and forceps, he was able to dissect and biopsy bilateral paratracheal and the subcarinal nodes. The procedure was initially performed in patients with confirmed bronchogenic carcinoma and either mediastinal widening on chest X-ray, or widening of the carinal angle at bronchoscopy. It was subsequently applied for biopsy of other causes of mediastinal lymphadenopathy including sarcoidosis, lymphosarcoma, and Hodgkin's disease. Carlens reported no complications in his first 100 patients. This procedure has since become standard in the preoperative staging of patients with suspected mediastinal nodal involvement and non-small cell lung cancer.

In circumstances of nondiagnostic cervical mediastinoscopy, exploratory thoracotomy remained necessary. In 1966, McNeill and Chamberlain[26] proposed an alternative procedure to bridge the gap between these extremes in the diagnostic armamentarium. They performed anterior mediastinotomy through the bed of the resected second costal cartilage to obtain tissue from hilar and mediastinal masses and to occasionally perform lung biopsy. They commented that this approach is particularly useful to obtain tissue before radiation therapy for an anterior mediastinal mass. "Chamberlain's procedure" is still useful for this indication today.

During the four decades between 1920 and 1960, the incidence of primary lung cancer increased logarithmically. Surgical experience with this disease process has demonstrated that mediastinal lymph node metastasis is the single most important prognostic indicator. Naruke and colleagues[27,28] performed careful pathologic examination of resected mediastinal nodes obtained at the time of pulmonary resection, and assigned these nodes to specific anatomic locations with numeric designations. This system has become the accepted international standard for mapping intrapulmonary, hilar, and mediastinal lymph nodes, and defines the nodal designation in the current staging system for non-small cell lung cancer.[29]

SUMMARY

One century ago, thoracic surgery was in its infancy. Since then, advances in chest radiology have allowed for reliable and early detection of thoracic ailments. Refinements in anesthesiology and surgical technique have led to the development of a plethora of techniques for the diagnosis, staging, and treatment of mediastinal disease. As the disease processes we encounter have expanded and evolved, so too has our surgical armamentarium.

REFERENCES

1. Meade RH. A history of thoracic surgery. Springfield (IL): Charles C. Thomas, Publisher; 1961.
2. Dalton ML, Connally SR. Median sternotomy. Surg Gynecol Obstet 1993;176(6):615–24.
3. Milton H. Mediastinal surgery. Lancet 1897;1:872–5.
4. Salem MR, Ylagan LB, Collins VJ. Historical note: the first successful removal of a mediastinal mass. Anesth Analg 1970;49(4):600–3.
5. Pearse HE. Mediastinitis following cervical suppuration. Ann Surg 1938;108(4):588–611.
6. Lilienthal H. Carcinoma of thoracic esophagus extrapleural resection and plastic. Ann Surg 1921; 74(3):259–79.
7. Harrington SW. The surgical treatment of mediastinal tumors. Ann Surg 1932;96(5):343–66.
8. Heuer GJ. Surgical treatment of tumors of the mediastinum. Ann Surg 1941;113(3):357–63.
9. Blades B. Mediastinal tumors. Ann Surg 1946; 123(5):749–64.
10. Sabiston DC, Scott HW. Primary neoplasms and cysts of the mediastinum. Ann Surg 1952;136(5): 777–97.
11. Wood MG, Hagen JA. Surgery of myasthenia gravis. In: Pearson FG, Cooper JD, editors. Thoracic surgery. 2nd edition. Philadelphia: Churchill Livingstone; 2002. p. 1624–35.
12. Blalock A, Mason MF, Morgan HJ, et al. Myasthenia gravis and tumors of the thymic region. Ann Surg 1939;110(4):544–61.
13. Kirby TJ, Ginsberg RJ. Transcervical thymectomy. In: Shields TW, Locicero J, editors. General thoracic surgery. 6th edition. Philadelphia: Lippincott, Williams, and Wilkins; 2005. p. 2634–7.
14. Blalock A. Thymectomy in the treatment of myasthenia gravis: report of twenty cases. J Thorac Cardiovasc Surg 1944;13:316–39.
15. Keynes G. Investigations into thymic disease and tumor formation. Br J Surg 1955;42(175):449–62.
16. Crile G. Thymectomy through the neck. Surgery 1964;59(2):213–5.
17. Carlens E, Johansson L, Olsson P. Mediastinoscopy auxiliary to thymectomy by the cervical route. Bronches 1967;17(5):408–10.
18. Kirschner PA, Osserman KE, Kark AE. Studies in myasthenia gravis-transcervical total thymectomy. JAMA 1969;209(6):906–10.
19. Cooper JD, Al-Jilaihawa AN, Pearson FG, et al. An improved technique to facilitate transcervical thymectomy for myasthenia gravis. Ann Thorac Surg 1988;45(3):242–7.

20. Calhoun RF, Ritter JH, Guthrie TJ, et al. Results of transcervical thymectomy for myasthenia gravis in 100 consecutive patients. Ann Surg 1999;230(4): 555–61.

21. Shrager JB, Nathan D, Brinster CJ, et al. Outcomes after 151 extended transcervical thymectomies for myasthenia gravis. Ann Thorac Surg 2006;82: 1863–9.

22. Daniels AC. A method of biopsy useful in diagnosing certain intrathoracic diseases. Chest 1949;16:360–7.

23. Harken DE, Black H, Clauss R, et al. A simple cervico-mediastinal exploration for tissue diagnosis of intrathoracic disease. N Engl J Med 1954;251(26):1041–4.

24. Rouviere H. Anatomy of the human lymphatic system. Ann Arbor (MI): Edwards; 1938. p. 318.

25. Carlens E. Mediastinoscopy: a method for inspection and tissue biopsy in the superior mediastinum. Chest 1959;36(4):343–52.

26. McNeill TM, Chamberlain JM. Diagnostic anterior mediastinotomy. Ann Thorac Surg 1966;2(4):532–9.

27. Naruke T, Suemasu K, Ishikawa S. Surgical treatment for lung cancer with metastasis to mediastinal lymph nodes. J Thorac Cardiovasc Surg 1976;71(2): 279–85.

28. Naruke T, Suemasu K, Ishikawa S. Lymph node mapping and curability at various levels of metastasis in resected lung cancer. J Thorac Cardiovasc Surg 1978;76(6):832–9.

29. Mountain CF. Revisions in the International system for staging lung cancer. Chest 1997;111(6):1710–7.

Utility of Positron Emission Tomography in the Mediastinum: Moving Beyond Lung and Esophageal Cancer Staging

Varun Puri, MD, Bryan F. Meyers, MD, MPH*

KEYWORDS

- PET • Mediastinum • Lymphoma • Thymoma
- Germ cell tumor

Broadly, all imaging can be divided into functional/molecular and anatomic. Functional imaging may be defined as the "in vivo characterization and measurement of biologic processes at the cellular and molecular level."[1] Positron emission tomography (PET) is the most widely employed functional imaging technique, while the modern-day prototype of anatomic imaging is the CT scan.

The last decade has seen a rapid increase in the use of PET technology in clinical medicine, and the trend is expected to continue (**Fig. 1**).

Much of this has been in the field of oncology, with PET being used to diagnose and stage tumors and to assess response to therapy, usually in conjunction with other imaging modalities.

TECHNICAL ASPECTS

PET is based upon a chemical process termed "annihilation," which involves the collision of an electron with a positron that is emitted by a radioisotope. The process results in the production of two photons that simultaneously move in diametrically opposite directions and are detected by a PET scanner that encircles the body. Several positron-emitting isotopes have been developed (**Table 1**), but 18F fluorodeoxyglucose (FDG) is

used most commonly because of its convenient half-life (110 minutes) and easy availability.

Lack of detailed resolution and inability to accurately localize anatomy on PET images have been the inherent drawbacks of PET technology. These weaknesses have led scientists to investigate the possibility of combining PET with the precise anatomic imaging offered by CT. Two dichotomous approaches have been pursued: software fusion and hardware fusion. Attempts to align or register CT and PET data sets by using fusion software have proven successful imaging the brain. In the remainder of the body, however, differences in scanner bed profiles, external patient positioning, and internal organ movement present challenges to the pure software approaches.[2] Hardware fusion has largely resolved these issues with the introduction of the combined PET/CT scanner. This technology has been commercially available since 2001 and most PET scanners in the United States are now combined CT/PET scanners. One must understand, however, that the CT scan performed as part of the CT/PET is usually a noncontrast study using a lower radiation dose and provides less anatomic detail than a contrast-enhanced standard CT scan, especially in the mediastinum. Other attempts at combining functional and

Division of Cardiothoracic Surgery, Washington University School of Medicine, Barnes- Jewish Hospital, Queeny Tower, 3108, One Barnes-Jewish Hospital Plaza, St. Louis, MO 63110, USA
* Corresponding author.
E-mail address: meyersb@wudosis.wustl.edu (B.F. Meyers).

Thorac Surg Clin 19 (2009) 7–15
doi:10.1016/j.thorsurg.2008.09.006

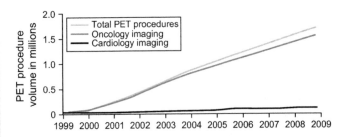

Fig. 1. Historic and forecast positron emission tomography (PET) procedure volume for cardiology and oncology from 1999 to 2009. (*Data from* Podoloff DA, Advani RJ, Allred C, et al. NCCN Task Force report: positron emission tomography (PET)/computed tomography (CT) scanning in cancer. J Natl Compr Canc Netw 2007;5(2):S1–22.)

anatomic imaging are ongoing and simultaneous PET-MRI scanning was reported recently.[3]

INTERPRETATION OF POSITRON EMISSION TOMOGRAPHY

FDG is the most commonly used tracer, and it delineates the uptake of glucose in various tissues of the body. Substitution of fluoride for a hydroxyl group allows cellular uptake but prevents metabolism of the tracer; thus tracer accumulation and activity are proportional to glycolysis in the anatomic area. Most tumors are obligate consumers of glucose and avidly accumulate FDG. Such uptake is also increased in various benign pathologies, such as inflammatory conditions, regenerating tissue in trauma, infection, persistent muscular activity, and granulomatous diseases. Familiarity with normal background activity in various tissues is essential in detecting abnormalities.

PET results are often reported with an SUV (standardized uptake value): a semi-quantitative measure of FDG uptake and activity in tissue that frequently has been criticized but also widely accepted because of its relative simplicity. The general formula for calculating SUV is activity per unit volume/injected activity/body weight. Maximum SUV is a better indicator than average SUV and provides more clinical information when the there is a large difference between the area of interest and background activity.

POSITRON EMISSION TOMOGRAPHY FOR THORACIC MALIGNANCIES

In the last decade, PET has been employed widely in the thorax in the diagnosis and follow-up of nonsmall cell lung cancer and esophageal cancer. For lung cancer, PET provides a significant advantage when combined with conventional anatomic imaging, in diagnosing and staging.[4] In a meta-analysis, PET was 95% sensitive and 77% specific in providing a diagnosis.[5] Similarly, for esophageal cancer, PET has been used in the diagnostic setting[6] and in monitoring response to treatment.[4] The discussion about PET in the thorax has been dominated by lung and esophageal malignancies because of the sheer number of papers and volume of information. For the purpose of this article, the authors will exclude the extensive and voluminous literature surrounding lung and esophageal cancer.

THE MEDIASTINUM

The mediastinum is populated by structures derived from all three germ lines with various basal metabolic rates. This unique anatomic and functional arrangement makes the mediastinum particularly suited to accurate evaluation with CT-PET. Myocardial and background mediastinal activity must be understood to accurately interpret PET imaging in this area. Mediastinal anatomy can be categorized along conventional lines[7] (**Fig. 2**), and this helps in classification of mediastinal pathology (**Box 1**).

The Anterior Mediastinum

Information about the use of PET in the anterior mediastinum is dominated by the application of PET to assessment of the thymus gland. FDG uptake is commonly seen in the thymus and can be

Table 1
Positron-emitting isotopes in clinical use

Positron Isotope	Half-Life (Minutes)	Use
F18	109.7	Metabolism, bone imaging
N13	9.96	Perfusion
C11	20.4	Multiple uses
Rb82	1.3	Perfusion
O15	2.07	Perfusion, blood flow, blood volume, metabolism

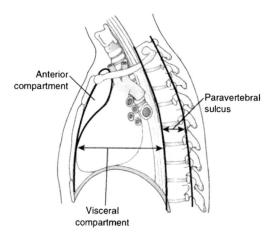

Fig. 2. Three-compartment model of mediastinal anatomy. (*From* Raymond DP, Daniel TM. Mediastinal anatomy and mediastinoscopy. In: Selke FW, del Nido PJ, Swanson SJ, editors. Sabiston and Spencer surgery of the chest. 7th edition. Philadelphia: Elsevier Saunders; 2005. p. 668; with permission.)

considered normal when there is no clinical, radiologic, or hematologic evidence of thymic pathology. It generally has been accepted that diffuse thymic FDG uptake is seen in more than half of prepubertal individuals and rapidly diminishes afterwards.[8] Subsequent studies, however, have shown that physiologic thymic uptake can be seen in patients well beyond puberty. One study examined thymic uptake of 18F-FDG PET in 94 patients ranging from 18 to 29 years of age and found that 32 of these patients exhibited physiologic thymic uptake.[9] Diffuse FDG uptake in the thymus does not discriminate normal from diseased thymus in the absence of other radiological or clinical information.

A study by Brink and colleagues[10] examined 18F-FDG PET findings in four sets of patients who had known malignancy: (1) children who had malignancy before chemotherapy, (2) children who had malignancy following chemotherapy, (3) adults who had lymphoma before chemotherapy, and (4) adults who had lymphoma following chemotherapy. The authors found increased 18F-FDG uptake in 73% of the children who had malignancy before chemotherapy and in 75% of the children who had malignancy following chemotherapy. They also found increased uptake in 5% of the adults who had lymphoma following chemotherapy, however. None of the adults who had lymphoma before chemotherapy exhibited increased thymic uptake. Thus, although thymic uptake is common in children, it occasionally may be seen in adults after chemotherapy, possibly related to an immunologic rebound.

The radiologic appearance of the so-called physiologic thymic uptake at PET is characteristic. It appears as a triangular retrosternal region of increased uptake. Although data are scant, when the SUVmax is greater than 4 in the thymus, this should not be considered physiologic or related to hyperplasia.[11] An uncommon scenario occurs when a patient who has a known thymic abnormality, often detected on a CT scan, undergoes PET to differentiate hyperplasia from neoplasia and, within neoplasia, to distinguish thymoma from thymic carcinoma. This is a clinical situation that occurs, but that does not have a large database of outcomes to offer guidance for decision making. Liu and colleagues[12] reported the preliminary findings of a small study with 10 cases of thymoma and two cases of thymic hyperplasia. The findings suggested diffuse uptake of FDG in thymic hyperplasia, confined focal uptake, in stage 1 and 2 thymomas, and multiple discrete foci of FDG uptake in stage 3 and 4 advanced invasive thymomas. Similarly, another small study showed that the pattern of uptake could predict hyperplasia versus thymoma in patients with myasthenia reliably.[13] Despite these small studies suggesting value in PET, it has not become standard practice to evaluate thymic neoplasia with PET.

The use of the semi-quantitative SUVmax can help differentiate between thymoma and thymic carcinoma, but PET has been inconsistent in distinguishing noninvasive from invasive thymoma (**Fig. 3**).

Sasaki and colleagues[14] found a mean SUV of 7.2 ± 2.9 for patients who had thymic carcinoma. This value was significantly greater than the values found for invasive thymoma (3.8 ± 1.3) and noninvasive thymoma (3.0 ± 1.0). By using an SUV of 5.0 as a cut-off, the authors achieved acceptable sensitivity (84.6%), specificity (92.3%), and accuracy (88.5%) in differentiating thymic carcinoma from thymoma. Given the relative rarity of thymic carcinoma, it seems likely that a similar sensitivity and specificity would be obtained with a purely clinical assessment based on CT scanning. They found no difference in SUV between invasive and noninvasive thymomas. An earlier study by Liu and colleagues,[12] however, indicated that PET may be able to distinguish invasive from noninvasive thymoma based upon pattern of FDG uptake. Kubota and colleagues[15] also showed that FDG uptake in invasive thymoma was significantly higher than in noninvasive thymoma. How that discrimination would be translated into a different treatment approach is not immediately clear.

In a retrospective review study group of eight patients, El Bawab and colleagues[13] found that FDG−PET was a very sensitive diagnostic tool in

---

Box 1
Mass lesions of the mediastinum

Anterior mediastinum
Neoplastic
Substernal goiter
Thymoma
Thymic hyperplasia
Thymic cyst
Ectopic parathyroid mass
Lymphoma
Teratoma
Germ cell tumor (GCT)
    Seminoma
    Nonnseminomatous GCT

Soft tissue tumor
Infectious/inflammatory
Mediastinitis
Vascular
Aneurysm of innominate vein
Superior vena cava aneurysm
Middle visceral mediastinum
Neoplastic
Tracheal tumors
Esophageal tumors
Lymphoma
Infectious/inflammatory
Fungal adenopathy
Sarcoidosis
Mycobacterial disease
Fibrosing mediastinitis
Mediastinitis
Cystic lesions
Bronchogenic
Esophageal
Pleuropericardial
Posterior paravertebral mediastinum
Neoplastic
Neurogenic tumors
    Neurofibroma
    Neurofibrosarcoma
    Ganglioneuroblastoma
    Parganglioma

Lymphoma
Soft tissue tumor
Infectious/inflammatory
Fungal adenopathy
Sarcoidosis
Mycobacterial disease
Fibrosing mediastinitis
Mediastinal abscess
Cystic lesions
Bronchogenic
Esophageal
Others
Extramedullary hematopoiesis

---

detecting residual, recurrent, and metastatic disease in patients after thymectomy for thymoma, but it was not superior to CT scan.

Lymphoma

Lymphoma represents less than 4% of all neoplasia but may account for up to 50% of PET scans performed at referral centers.[1] Lymphoma can involve any organ system and mimic other tumors in its radiologic appearance. The mediastinum may be the primary site of disease, like in Hodgkins's lymphoma and primary mediastinal B cell lymphoma, or it may be involved as part of systemic disease.

Like all malignancies, the diagnosis of lymphoma requires histologic assessment, and PET is not likely to be used as an initial diagnostic modality. Routine staging of a biopsy- established lymphoma involves a CT scan with contrast, from the neck to the pelvis, and a PET scan in addition. PET virtually has replaced gallium scan in the pretreatment work-up of lymphoma. A health technology assessment report from the United Kingdom[4] summarized that PET was 90% sensitive and 90% specific when used in the initial staging of lymphoma. They also noted that the addition of PET changed the staging/management in up to 20% of patients. One caveat was that staging PET scan can be omitted as part of staging when management is to consist of observation alone, like in some patients who have follicular lymphoma. The International Harmonization Project has provided guidelines for the use of PET in lymphoma.[16] They recommend that a pretherapy baseline PET is not obligatory for assessing response after treatment of patients who have some subgroups of lymphoma, because these

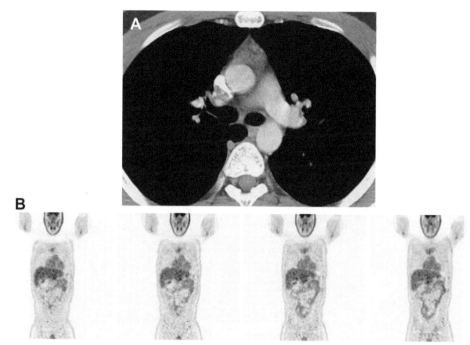

Fig. 3. A 33-year-old woman with stage IIa thymoma (case 9). (*A*) Axial CT shows solid homogenous mass in the anterior mediastinum. (*B*) 18F fluorodeoxyglucose (FDG)—positron emission tomography shows intense FDG uptake in the anterior mediastinum and contiguous pleura suggesting thymoma. (*From* El-Bawab H, Al-Sugair AA, Rafay M, et al. Role of flourine-18 fluorodeoxyglucose positron emission tomography in thymic pathology. Euro J Cardiothorac Surg 2007;31(4):734; with permission.)

lymphomas routinely are FDG-avid. Pretherapy PET, however, may be valuable, because it can facilitate the interpretation of post-therapy PET.

PET has had the highest impact in management of lymphoma in the assessment of response to therapy and guiding decisions about further treatment (**Fig. 4**). Juweid and colleagues[17] assessed response to therapy in 54 patients who had aggressive non-Hodgkin's lymphoma using the established criteria in conjunction with PET scan results and compared response with progression-free survival. Using the CT-based criteria alone, 17 patients experienced a complete response, and seven experienced a less than complete response. In contrast, when PET results were incorporated, 35 patients experienced a complete response, and no patients experienced less-than-complete response. Therefore, a negative PET scan even in the presence of a residual mass was interpreted correctly as a complete response. Subsequently, the International Harmonization Project has published revised response criteria for treating lymphoma incorporating PET.[18]

Post-therapy inflammatory changes can be seen after chemotherapy and radiation. To minimize the frequency of these changes, which potentially confound the interpretation of PET scans, the International Harmonization Project recommends that scans should not be performed sooner than 3 weeks after chemotherapy and should preferably occur 8 to 12 weeks after completion of radiotherapy. Response assessment at the conclusion of therapy is recommended; however, no specific guidelines about midtherapy assessment are available. Visual assessment alone appears to be adequate for determining whether PET is positive or negative at the conclusion of therapy, and quantitative or semiquantitative approaches (eg, using the SUV) do not seem necessary.[16]

The true incidence of false-positive scans in follow-up, however, remains unresolved. Zinzani and colleagues[19] followed 151 patients who had mediastinal lymphoma (57 with Hodgkin's disease and 94 with aggressive non-Hodgkin's lymphoma after the end of front-line treatment. Patients who had a positive PET scan of the mediastinum underwent CT scanning and surgical biopsy. In 30 cases, a suspicion of lymphoma relapse was raised based on positive mediastinal PET scanning. Histology confirmed this suspicion in 17 out of 30 patients, whereas either benign (nine fibrosis, three sarcoid-like granulomatosis) or unrelated neoplastic conditions (one thymoma) were demonstrated in

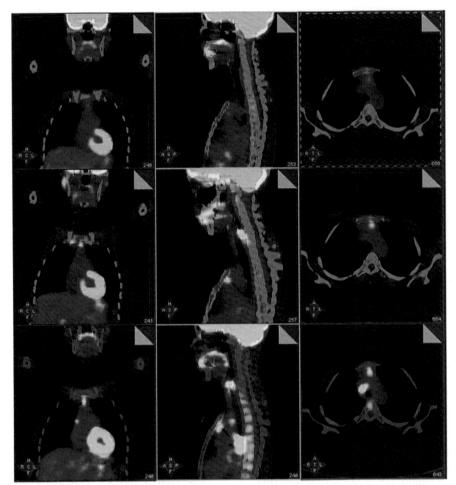

Fig. 4. Positron emission tomography (PET)-positive residual mass in a patient with initial diagnosis of stage IIA nodular sclerosis Hodgkin's disease. This patient underwent a restaging PET/ CT scan 2 months after treatment with six cycles of doxorubicin, bleomycin, vinblastine, and dacarbazine. (*Top panel*) Fused PET/CT images show increased uptake clearly greater than that of mediastinal blood pool structures within the residual anterior mediastinal mass, consistent with persistent disease. (*Middle panel*) A follow-up PET/CT scan performed 2 months later shows substantially more intense uptake in the same area, again suggesting persistent disease. (*Lower panel*) A third follow-up scan performed 4 months thereafter also demonstrates intense uptake in the same area but now with additional new sites of disease in the right paratracheal, right hilar, and subcarinal regions, indicating frank disease progression. The patient then underwent high-dose chemotherapy and autologous stem cell transplantation. (*Courtesy of* M. Juweid, MD, Iowa City, IA.)

the remaining 13 patients (43%). SUVmax was significantly higher among the 17 patients who had signs of relapse (median 5.95, range 3.5 to 26.9) than among the 13 patients who stayed in remission (median 2.90, range 1.4 to 3.3). They recommended routine biopsy before further therapy in this setting.

In addition, PET is useful for directing biopsy of the most suspicious areas based on SUV.[1]

Germ Cell Tumors

Mediastinal germ cell tumors are uncommon tumors that occur predominantly within the anterior mediastinum and frequently present as a very large mass with local compression. The mediastinum can also be involved by metastatic germ cell tumor from the gonads. Chest CT and evaluation of serum tumor markers provide the critical workup before tissue diagnosis is obtained. PET has found a niche in the evaluation of these metabolically active tumors.

Seminomas are extremely sensitive to chemotherapy and radiation and primarily are treated nonsurgically. The dilemma lies in managing postchemotherapy residual masses. Traditionally, masses larger than 3 cm on CT have been considered to potentially harbor residual disease and thus offered further therapy, usually resection. This approach was re-evaluated with addition of FDG PET studies in patients with metastatic pure seminoma who had radiographically defined post-chemotherapy residual masses.[20] The PET studies were correlated with either the histology of the resected lesion or the clinical outcome documented by CT, tumor markers, or physical examination during follow-up. All 19 cases with residual lesions greater than 3 cm and 35 (95%) of 37 with residual lesions less than or equal to 3 cm were predicted correctly by FDG PET. FDG-PET was superior to CT scan in detecting residual disease (specificity 100% versus 74%, sensitivity 80% versus 70%, positive predictive value 100% versus 37%, and negative predictive value 96% versus 92%, respectively).

In another report, FDG PET was shown to be accurate in the initial staging of germ cell tumors and in detecting unsuspected metastatic disease.[21]

Residual masses in nonseminomatous germ cell tumors (NSGCT) may contain necrotic tissue, viable NSGCT, or teratoma. Kollmannsberger and colleagues[22] studied patients who had NSGCT; independent reviewers who were blinded to each other's results evaluated the PET results and corresponding CT scan and tumor marker results in 85 residual lesions from 45 patients. Resulting sensitivities and specificities for the prediction of residual mass viability were as follows: PET, 59% sensitivity and 92% specificity; radiologic monitoring, 55% sensitivity and 86% specificity; and tumor markers (TUM), 42% sensitivity and 100% specificity. The positive and negative predictive values for PET were 91% and 62%, respectively. This study shows that a positive PET image after treatment was a strong predictor for the presence of viable carcinoma/teratoma. Conversely, a negative PET after the end of treatment does not allow one to avoid surgery, because 37% of all negative PET masses either progressed during 6 months of follow-up, or led to a histologic examination showing mature teratoma.

Only anecdotal reports show the usefulness of PET in mediastinal germ cell tumors,[23,24] but the identical biologic nature of disease in the mediastinum and elsewhere makes extrapolation from previous reports meaningful.

PARATHYROID ADENOMA

The incidence of mediastinal parathyroid glands requiring surgery was 3% in a large database.[25] Strategies to localize parathyroid tissue before parathyroid surgery encompass CT, MRI, 99Tc Sestamibi scan, ultrasound, arteriography, selective venous sampling, and FDG PET and 11C methionine PET. Beggs and colleagues[26] retrospectively evaluated 51 patients presenting with hyperparathyroidism, in whom other imaging techniques had failed to definitely identify the site of suspected parathyroid adenoma. All patients had undergone 11C methionine PET scanning. Patients were followed up by surgical histology, or clinically if surgery was not performed. 11C methionine PET scanning was found to have a sensitivity of 83%, a specificity of 100%, and an accuracy of 88% in successfully locating parathyroid adenomas. Most false negatives were caused by adenomas in the lower mediastinum that were outside the area of scanning.

Middle Mediastinum

Lymphoma, once again, is a prominent differential diagnosis in middle mediastinal neoplasia. Inflammatory involvement of mediastinal lymph nodes (LNs) may be acute, subacute, or chronic. Acute lymphadenopathy, often related to pneumonia, is FDG-avid, but the activity diminishes with follow-up studies. Subacute or chronic LN involvement may be fungal or mycobacterial. Mediastinal histoplasmosis is a frequently seen entity in the midwestern United States and can masquerade as a malignant mediastinal process in patients who have known malignancy elsewhere.[27] The presence of calcification in LNs on CT and concomitant granulomas in the lungs may provide a clue to diagnosis, but tissue diagnosis frequently is required.

The assessment of mediastinal LNs with PET is even more problematic in tuberculosis-endemic countries. In a study from Korea involving 674 patients who had lung cancer,[28] nodes with greater FDG uptake than the mediastinum at PET without benign pattern calcification or high attenuation (greater than 70 Hounsfield units) on unenhanced CT scans were regarded as being positive for malignancy. The overall sensitivity, specificity, and accuracy of PET/CT for mediastinal nodal staging were 61%, 96%, and 86%, respectively. The high specificity was achieved at the expense of sensitivity by interpreting calcified nodes or nodes with high attenuation at CT, even with high FDG uptake at PET, as benign.

One scientist's false positive is another's true positive. Although sarcoidosis and other granulomatous lesions of the mediastinum can create a dilemma on PET imaging in patients who have known malignancy, scientists have found a unique application for PET in assessment of sarcoidosis. FDG uptake in sarcoidosis is nonspecific in both intensity and pattern, and it is not useful in making an initial diagnosis. Diffuse metastatic disease and lymphoma need to be ruled out. FDG uptake, however, can decrease when sarcoidosis is treated, and PET might be useful in monitoring the effectiveness of therapy.[29]

Brown adipose tissue can be variably FDG-avid. PET/CT scans were obtained in a study of 845 patients who had known cancer.[30] Fifteen patients (1.8%) who had focal hypermetabolic mediastinal brown fat were identified. Hypermetabolic mediastinal brown fat (mean SUVmax 5.7) was more common in children (four of eight) than in adults 11 of 837) and more common in women (9 of 372) than in men (2 of 465). Foci of hypermetabolic brown fat were localized to the paratracheal, paraesophageal, prevascular, and pericardial regions; interatrial septum; and azygoesophageal recess. Ten patients also had extramediastinal hypermetabolic brown fat in the neck, thorax, and abdomen. The authors concluded that precise localization of brown fat with fusion PET/CT is important in preventing misinterpretation as malignancy. Premedication with diazepam and fentanyl has been used to suppress FDG uptake in brown fat.[31]

Posterior Mediastinum

Cystic lesions arising from the foregut are not FDG-avid. Neurogenic tumors are the most common mass lesions unique to the posterior mediastinum. Schwannomas are benign peripheral nerve sheath tumors than can arise from intercostal nerves. Studies have tried to differentiate schwannomas from sarcoma preoperatively based on PET. Although a cutoff SUVmax of 1.8 has been proposed,[32] subsequent studies[33,34] have shown significantly higher SUVmax in benign schwannomas, and the diagnosis must be considered despite high FDG avidity. Neurofibrosarcomas of the posterior mediastinum, like sarcomas elsewhere, are expected to have significant FDG avidity.

SUMMARY

PET and PET-CT are rapidly evolving as modalities of thoracic imaging. In the mediastinum, PET can provide information to distinguish thymic hyperplasia from neoplasia, although the use of this imaging for this purpose is not accepted uniformly as necessary. PET is the standard of care in staging and follow-up of mediastinal lymphoma and in follow-up of metastatic seminomas after chemotherapy. Mycobacterial/fungal infections, sarcoidosis, and brown fat can mimic malignant findings on PET in the mediastinum.

REFERENCES

1. Podoloff DA, Advani RJ, Allred C, et al. NCCN task force report: positron emission tomography (PET)/computed tomography (CT) scanning in cancer. J Natl Compr Canc Netw 2007;5(2):S1–22.
2. Blodgett TM, Meltzer CC, Townsend DW. PET/CT: form and function. Radiology 2007;242(2):360–85.
3. Judenhofer MS, Wehrl HF, Newport DF, et al. Simultaneous PET-MRI: a new approach for functional and morphological imaging. Nat Med 2008;14(4):459–65.
4. Facey K, Bradbury I, Laking G, et al. Overview of the clinical effectiveness of positron emission tomography imaging in selected cancers. Health Technol Assess 2007;11(44):1–285.
5. Gould MK, Maclean CC, Kuschner WG, et al. Accuracy of positron emission tomography for diagnosis of pulmonary nodules and mass lesions: a meta-analysis. JAMA 2001;285(7):914–24.
6. Meyers BF, Downey RJ, Decker PA, et al. The utility of positron emission tomography in staging of potentially operable carcinoma of the thoracic esophagus: results of the American College of Surgeons Oncology Group Z0060 trial. J Thorac Cardiovasc Surg 2007;133(3):738–45.
7. Raymond DP, Daniel TM. Mediastinal anatomy and mediastinoscopy. In: Selke FW, delNido PJ, Swanson SJ, editors. Sabiston and Spencer surgery of the chest. 7th edition. Philadelphia: Elsevier Saunders; 2005. p. 657–66.
8. Patel PM, Alibazoglu H, Ali A, et al. Normal thymic uptake of FDG on PET imaging. Clin Nucl Med 1996;21(10):772–5.
9. Nakahara T, Fujii H, Ide M, et al. FDG uptake in the morphologically normal thymus: comparison of FDG positron emission tomography and CT. Br J Radiol 2001;74(885):821–4.
10. Brink I, Reinhardt MJ, Hoegerle S, et al. Increased metabolic activity in the thymus studied with FDG PET: age dependency and frequency after chemotherapy. J Nucl Med 2001;42(4):591–5.
11. Fernidand B, Gupta P, Kramer EL. Spectrum of thymic uptake at 18F-FDG PET. Radiographics 2004;24(6):1611–6.
12. Liu RS, Yeh SH, Huang MH, et al. Use of fluorine-18 fluorodeoxyglucose positron emission tomography in the detection of thymoma: a preliminary report. Eur J Nucl Med 1995;22(12):1402–7.
13. El-Bawab H, Al-Sugair AA, Rafay M, et al. Role of flourine-18 fluorodeoxyglucose positron emission tomography in thymic pathology. Eur J Cardiothorac Surg 2007;31(4):731–6.
14. Sasaki M, Kuwabara Y, Ichiya Y, et al. Differential diagnosis of thymic tumors using a combination of 11C-methionine PET and FDG PET. J Nucl Med 1999;40(10):1595–601.

15. Kubota K, Yamada S, Kondo T, et al. PET imaging of primary mediastinal tumours. Br J Cancer 1996; 73(7):882–6.

16. Juweid ME, Stroobnts S, Hoekstra OS, et al. Use of positron emission tomography for response assessment of lymphoma: consensus of the imaging subcommittee of international harmonization project in lymphoma. J Clin Oncol 2007;25(5):571–8.

17. Juweid ME, Wiseman ME, Vose JM, et al. Response assessment of aggressive non-Hodgkin's lymphoma by integrated International Workshop Criteria and fluorine-18-fluorodeoxyglucose positron emission tomography. J Clin Oncol 2005;23(21):4652–61.

18. Cheson BD, Pfistner B, Juweid ME, et al. Revised response criteria for malignant lymphoma. J Clin Oncol 2007;25(5):579–86.

19. Zinzani PL, Tani M, Trisolini R, et al. Histological verification of positive positron emission tomography findings in the follow-up of patients with mediastinal lymphoma. Haematologica 2007;92(6):771–7.

20. deSantis M, Becherer A, Bokemeyer C, et al. 18fluoro-deoxy-D-glucose positron emission tomography is a reliable predictor for viable tumor in postchemotherapy seminoma: an update of the prospective multicentric SEMPET trial. J Clin Oncol 2004;22(6):1034–9.

21. Hain S, O'Doherty M, Timothy A, et al. Fluorodeoxyglucose PET in the initial staging of germ cell tumours. Eur J Nucl Med 2000;27(5):590–4.

22. Kollmannsberger C, Oeschle K, Dohmen B, et al. Prospective comparison of [18F]fluorodeoxyglucose positron emission tomography with conventional assessment by computed tomography scans and serum tumor markers for the evaluation of residual masses in patients with nonseminomatous germ cell carcinoma. Cancer 2002;94(9):2353–62.

23. Bachman J, Ernestus K, Werner T, et al. Detection of primary choriocarcinoma in the mediastinum by F-18 FDG positron emission tomography. Clin Nucl Med 2007;32(8):663–5.

24. Aide N. Enlarging residual mass after treatment of a nonseminomatous germ cell tumor: growing teratoma syndrome or cancer recurrence? J Clin Oncol 2007;25(28):4494–6.

25. Nilubol N, Beyer T, Prinz RA, et al. Mediastinal hyperfunctioning parathyroids: incidence, evolving treatment, and outcome. Am J Surg 2007;194(1):53–6.

26. Beggs AD, Hain SF. Localization of parathyroid adenomas using 11C-methionine positron emission tomography. Nucl Med Commun 2005;26(2):133–6.

27. Mackie GC, Pohlen JM. Mediastinal histoplasmosis: F-18 FDG PET and CT findings simulating malignant disease. Clin Nucl Med 2005;30(9):633–5.

28. Kim YK, Lee KS, Kim BT, et al. Mediastinal nodal staging of nonsmall cell lung cancer using integrated 18F-FDG PET/CT in a tuberculosis-endemic country: diagnostic efficacy in 674 patients. Cancer 2007;109(6):1068–77.

29. Nishiyama Y, Yamamoto Y, Fukunaga K, et al. Comparative evaluation of 18F–FDG PET and 67Ga scintigraphy in patients with sarcoidosis. J Nucl Med 2006;47(10):1571–6.

30. Truong MT, Erasmus JJ, Munden RF, et al. Focal FDG uptake in mediastinal brown fat mimicking malignancy: a potential pitfall resolved on PET/CT. Am J Roentgenol 2004;183(4):1127–32.

31. Gelfand MJ, O'hara SM, Curtwright LA, et al. Premedication to block [(18)F]FDG uptake in the brown adipose tissue of pediatric and adolescent patients. Pediatr Radiol 2005;35(10):984–90.

32. Watanabe H, Shinozaki T, Aoki J, et al. Glucose metabolic analysis of musculoskeletal tumors using fluorine-18-FDG PET as an aid in preoperative planning. J Bone Joint Surg Br 2000;82(5):760–7.

33. Ahmed AR, Watanabe H, Aoki J, et al. Schwannoma of the extremities: the role of PET in preoperative planning. Eur J Nucl Med 2001;28(10):1541–51.

34. Beaulieu S, Rubin B, Djang D, et al. Positron emission tomography of schwannomas: emphasizing its potential in preoperative planning. Am J Roentgenol 2004;182(4):971–4.

Genetic Markers of Mediastinal Tumors

Matthew D. Taylor, MD[a], David R. Jones, MD[b],*

KEYWORDS

- Mediastinal tumors • Genetic markers • Thymoma
- Germ cell tumors • Lymphoma • Neurogenic tumors

Most mediastinal tumors are represented by thymomas, lymphomas, germ cell tumors, and neurogenic tumors. Pathologic staging remains the cornerstone in determining the prognosis for malignant mediastinal tumors. The rise in molecular pathologic techniques now permits the investigation of the genetic basis of these tumors to obtain further insight into the gene products responsible for their development and progression.

The purpose of this article is to review the genetic markers and chromosomal aberrations that have been uncovered for the more common mediastinal tumors seen by thoracic surgeons. It discusses the association of genetic markers with thymoma, thymic carcinoma, germ cell tumors, lymphoma, and neurogenic tumors.

THYMOMA / THYMIC CARCINOMA

Thymoma, a neoplasm of thymic epithelial cells, is the most common primary tumor of the anterior mediastinum in adults between the ages of 40 and 60.[1] Thymomas are a heterogenous group of tumors that traditionally have an indolent course; however, they maintain the capacity to invade surrounding structures and metastasize. The World Health Organization (WHO) thymoma classification scheme (1999) was updated in 2004 and has been shown to be an independent prognostic indicator in patients who have thymomas.[2] The WHO thymoma classification with comparison to the classical clinicopathological and histogenic classification is depicted in **Table 1**.

Initial studies have investigated the chromosomal abnormalities associated with the development of the rare, thymocyte-poor WHO types A, B3, and C. Zettl and colleagues[3] investigated genetic aberrations in 37 thymoma patients. In this study, 12 patients had WHO type A thymomas; 16 had WHO type B3 thymomas, and 9 had WHO type C thymomas. Genetic alterations were analyzed by comparative genomic hybridization and fluorescent in situ hybridization (FISH). In the type A thymomas, 11 of 12 tumors showed no chromosomal gain or loss, while one specimen demonstrated a partial loss of the short arm of chromosome 6.

Contrasting these results, all B3 thymomas showed evidence of chromosomal imbalance. Of the 16 B3 thymomas investigated, gain in chromosome 1q was the most frequent genetic aberration, found in 67% of specimens. Gain in chromosome 1 has been linked to other human cancers.[4] Loss of chromosome 13q occurred in five specimens (31%). Chromosome 13q contains the tumor suppressor genes RB1 and BRCA2.[5]

Loss of chromosome 6 was found in six B3 specimens (38%). Chromosome 6p has attracted interest, as it contains the human leukocyte antigen (HLA) gene, suggesting that abnormalities of chromosome 6 may cause loss of the protective capacities of the HLA molecules. This could lead to the formation of a population of T cells aggressively targeting self-antigens, which may lead to paraneoplastic autoimmune diseases associated with thymomas.[3,6] Other investigators have confirmed the importance of chromosomal aberration in chromosome 6 in association with tumor suppressor gene function and the development of breast[7] and colorectal cancer.[8]

a Department of Surgery, University of Virginia, Box 801359, Charlottesville, VA 22908, USA
b General Thoracic Surgery, Department of Surgery, University of Virginia, Box 800679, Charlottesville, VA 22908, USA
* Corresponding author.
E-mail address: djones@virginia.edu (D.R. Jones).

Thorac Surg Clin 19 (2009) 17–27
doi:10.1016/j.thorsurg.2008.09.004

Table 1
Classification of thymic tumors

Clinicopathological Classification	World Health Organization Type	Histogenetic Classification
Benign thymoma[a]	A	Medullary thymoma
	AB	Mixed thymoma
Malignant thymomas, category 1	B1	Predominantly cortical thymoma
	B2	Cortical thymoma
	B3	Well-differentiated thymic carcinoma
Malignant thymomas, category 2	C	Epidermoid keratinizing (squamous cell) carcinoma
		Epidermoid nonkeratinizing carcinoma
		Lymphoepithelioma-like carcinoma
		Sarcomatoid carcinoma (carcinosarcoma)
		Clear cell carcinoma
		Basaloid carcinoma
		Mucoepidermoid carcinoma
		Undifferentiated carcinoma

[a] The benign category is modified according to the postulate that type A and AB thymomas are clinically benign irrespective of invasiveness. Originally, all encapsulated thymomas were considered to be benign irrespective of their histology.

Data from Zhou R, Zettl A, Strobel P, et al. Thymic epithelial tumors can develop along two different pathogenetic pathways. Am J Pathol 2001;159:1854.

In type C thymoma specimens, chromosomal gain was found in 1q (56%), 17q (33%), and chromosome 18 (33%). Sixty-seven percent of type C thymomas had loss of chromosome 16q. Chromosome 16q contains several tumor suppressor genes, including RB2/p130[9] and cadherin genes CDH1, CDH8, and CDH13.[10] Loss of chromosome 6 (44%) and 3p and 17p (33%) also was found in type C thymomas.

Subsequent investigation of genetic alterations associated with thymomas suggests that these tumors develop along pathogenetic pathways characterized by 6q23.3–25.3 and the adenomatosis polyposis coli tumor suppressor gene at locus 5q21.[11] Genetic aberration of 5q21 is associated with genetic abnormalities of the p53 gene (17p13.1) and retinoblastoma gene (13q14). Thymomas of all WHO types had a 6q23.3–25.3 deletion. In contrast, no type A patients had deletion of the APC tumor suppressor gene locus at 5q21 or aberrations of the RB or p53 gene locus. The authors suggest that the absence of these aberrations in type A thymomas may be the reason for their benign behavior compared with type B3 or type C thymomas.

A robust genetic analysis of thymomas has been limited by the abundant non-neoplastic lymphocytes present in up to 70% of cases.[12] Inoue and colleagues were able to characterize the more common WHO type AB, B2, and B3 using microdissection and short-term primary culture of neoplastic thymic epithelial cells in 57 patients. Irrespective of WHO classification, loss of heterozygosity at chromosome 6 was found in 43% of specimens. Allelic imbalances were frequent at the locus of the retinoblastoma gene (13q14.3) and the E-cadherin gene (16q22.10). Furthermore, the presence of stage 4 thymic carcinoma was found to correlate with loss of heterozygosity of CDH1, the E-cadherin gene. Numerous other studies have demonstrated that reduced E-cadherin expression may impair tumor cell adhesion and result in metastasis.[13–15]

Recently, Lee and colleagues conducted a study of 39 thymomas representing WHO subtypes A, AB, B1, B2, and B3 of tumors using cDNA microarray technology.[16] Gene cluster analysis between WHO type A and type B3 found 70 genes that exhibited a different gene copy number between the two types of thymoma. **Table 2** illustrates the list of distinctive genes between type A and B3. Cluster analysis between the three subgroups, including type A, type B1+B2, and type B3 was performed and is shown in **Table 3**. The authors conclude that thymomas may be divided into four genetically distinct groups, A, AB, B1+ B2, and B3. Such an analysis may provide insight into potential candidate genes for biomarkers of thymic disease.

A particularly aggressive poorly differentiated thymic carcinoma has been associated with a highly specific chromosomal rearrangement characterized by a three-way translocation of chromosomes 11, 15, and 19.[17] This particular chromosomal rearrangement is found in younger patients and carries a dismal prognostic outcome.[17]

In summary, molecular pathologic techniques have been able to distinguish chromosomal aberrations common to subtypes of thymomas. This chromosomal analysis has provided insight into the genes responsible for the pathogenesis of thymomas. Furthermore, gene cluster analysis of thymomas has further distinguished the differential gene expression patterns between subtypes, thereby correlating gene expression to histologic features of thymomas.

GERM CELL TUMORS
Seminoma

Mediastinal seminoma represents 3% to 4% of all neoplasms found in the mediastinum.[18] Discrepancies in the genetic alterations of mediastinal seminomas compared with gonadal seminomas has raised the question as to whether diagnostic criteria for gonadal seminoma is applicable to mediastinal seminoma work-up.[19,20] Accurate diagnosis of this germ cell tumor is critical because of a favorable response to chemotherapy and/or radiation. Genetic analysis of mediastinal seminomatous tumors has provided an improved understanding of the pathogenesis of this disease process.

Sung and colleagues[21] evaluated 23 cases of primary mediastinal seminoma using immunohistochemistry and FISH. Chromosomal analysis uncovered the presence of chromosome 12 abnormalities in 96% of mediastinal seminoma specimens, with 87% resulting in 12p overexpression. Immunohistochemical analysis was performed using antibodies to OCT4, c-kit, placental-like alkaline phosphatase, CD30, and a panel of cytokeratins. OCT4 is a transcriptional factor regulating pluripotency in germ cells and stem cells and has been found to be a sensitive marker for detecting seminomas. The combination of intense nuclear staining with OCT4 and 12p chromosomal abnormalities in mediastinal seminomas may add significant diagnostic utility to the diagnosis of mediastinal seminomas.

Nonseminomatous Germ Cell Tumors

Studies focused on the genetic markers of nonseminomatous primary mediastinal tumors are limited. Teratomas are the most common type of mediastinal germ cell tumor. They contain two or more embryo embryonic layers represented by the ectoderm, mesoderm, and endoderm. Hiroshima and colleagues compared genetic markers of apoptosis and proliferative activity by means of immunohistochemical analysis of Bcl-2, Bax, p53, and α-fetoprotein in mature and immature teratomas of the mediastinum.[22] This study concluded that mature teratomas have overexpression of p53, which is related to the higher apoptotic index observed than in immature teratomas. In contrast, immature teratomas exhibited lower rates of apoptosis but higher proliferative activity. These observations may explain the clinical aggressive nature of immature teratomas compared with mature teratomas of the mediastinum.

There are limited data on the genetic markers of embryonic and yolk sac germ cell tumors. The most common chromosomal abnormality found in these germ cell tumors, however, is an increased copy number of chromosome 12p usually in the form of an isochromosome.[23,24]

Genetic Markers to Predict Germ Cell Tumor Response to Chemotherapy

There is evidence that the presence of an isochromosome of the short arm of chromosome 12 (i(12p)) in germ cell tumors is associated with a poor response to chemotherapeutic agents.[25] Among patients with this karyotypic abnormality, 75% of patients required resection for residual disease following chemotherapy as compared with 19% of patients without the abnormality. Furthermore, the presence of the i(12p) was found in 80% of the patients who died from their disease. This suggests an important role of chromosome 12p in the pathogenesis of germ cell tumors and their response to chemotherapy.

LYMPHOMA

Mediastinal lymphomas are derived from either mediastinal lymph nodes or the thymus gland. Lymphoma derived from mediastinal lymph nodes represents a wide spectrum of systemic nodal lymphoma and are beyond the scope of this article. The authors focus their discussion on the subtypes of mediastinal lymphoma of thymic origin.

Primary Mediastinal B-cell Lymphoma

Primary mediastinal B-cell lymphoma (PMBL) is a lymphoma derived from thymic medullary B cells.[26] It represents 2% to 3% of non-Hodgkin's lymphomas and primarily affects young adults in their third and fourth decade.[27] PMBL is distinguished from diffuse large B-cell lymphomas by

Table 2
Distinctive gene between types A and B3 thymomas

Identification No.	Symbol	Cytoband	Name	Type A Gain	Type A Loss	Type B3 Gain	Type B3 Loss
AA186327	SNX14	6q14-q15	Sorting nexin 14				5/8
AA458945	RAB30	11q12-q14	RAB3member RAS oncogene family	5/6			4/8
A1201652	EST			4/6		1/8	3/8
A1337344	HSRGI	16q23.1	HSV-1 stimubtion-related gene 1	6/6		3/8	1/8
AA991868	EST			6/6		3/8	2/8
AA465687	HCC-4	2q24.2	Cervical cancer oncogene 4	6/6		2/8	4/8
A1493835	ESTs			6/6		2/8	1/8
AW087220	ESTs			4/6			
AA478436	SMARCD2	17q23-q24	SWI/SNF-related, matrix- associated, actin-dependent regulator of chromatin, subfamily d, member 2	6/6			2/8
A1015542	TG737	13q12.1	Probe hTg737	5/6		2/8	
A1733279	ESTs			6/6		2/8	4/8
AA973681	ESTs			3/6			
N93021	TBCA	5q14.1					5/8
AA917489	ESTs			6/6			
AA775364	RPL30	8q22	Ribosomal protein L30	1/6			
AA987488	ESTs			2/6			2/8
AA478585	BTN3A3	6q23-q24	Butyrophilin, subfamily 3, member A3	1/6			2/8
A1291184	OCLN	13q12.1	Occludin	5/6			2/8
A1348521	HBSIL	6q23-q24	HBSI-like				6/8
AA287917	TNPOI	5q13.2	Karyopherin (importin) beta 2	2/6			2/8
AA885609	MAPIA	15q13-qter	Microtubule-associated protein IA				8/8
A1375415	ESTs						2/8
AA489670	ESTs						3/8
A1972677	MSMB	10q11.2	Microseminorotein, beta	1/6			1/6
N71628	SPIB	19q13.3-q13.4	Spi-B transcription factor (Spi-I/PU.I-related)	3/5			1/6
A1383789	ESTs			2/6			3/8
A1261862	ESTs			2/6			
A1985214	TFPI	2q31-q32.1	Tissue factor pathway				
H17513	HSPAIL	6p25-p24	Heat shock 70kDa protein I-like				2/8
T61428	NEDD9	2q12-qter	Neural precursor cell- expressed, developmentally down-regulated 9	2/6			2/8
N90109	NCL	Xq22.1	Nucleolin	3/6			1/8
A1972568	RPL36A	3p21	Ribosomal protein L36a	3/6			
AA442092	CTNNBI		Catenin, beta I, 88kDa				1/8
AA902196	ESTs			2/6			1/8
AW009090	NDUFB3	2q31.3	NADH dehydrogenase I beta subcomplex, 3, 12dDa				1/8
AA975250	MAT28	5q34-q35.1	Methionine adenosyltransferase ii, beta				3/8
A1281237	C13orf12	13q12.3	Chromosome 13 open reading frame 12				3/8

(continued on next page)

Table 2
(continued)

Identification No.	Symbol	Cytoband	Name	Type A Gain	Type A Loss	Type B3 Gain	Type B3 Loss
H51066	OBRGRP	1p31.3	Leptin receptor gene-related protein				2/8
AA465386	DDX21		DEAD (Asp-Glu-Ala-Asp) box polypeptide 21				3/8
A1951501	RPL12	9q34	Ribosomal protein L12	6/6		1/8	
AW075424	SFRS3	6p21	Splicing factor, arginine/serine-rich3	6/6			1/8
A1086414	EST						2/8
A1279626	EST						2/8
AA677257	TPMT	6p22.3	Thiopurine S-methyltransferase				6/8
AA887201	C13orf1	13q14	Chromosome 13 open reading frame I				1/8
A1284218	ESTs			2/6			1/8
AA991871	FOXAI	14q12-q13	Forkhead box AI	3/6			
AA864434	ESTs			4/6		1/8	1/8
A1318162	FLJI4936	1p33-p32.1	Hypothetical protein FLJI4936				1/8
AA504351	ZNF146		Zinc finger protein 146		1/6		6/8
A1302566	ESTs			3/6			1/8
A1311303	ESTs						3/8
AW078798	UBB	17p12-p11.2	Ubiquitin B	6/6	2/6		
AA927666	ARCH	1p35.1	Archease	3/6			1/8
AA426027	SNX3	6q21	Sorting nexin 3	3/6			6/8
A1262055	ESTs						1/8
AA936514	C6orf10	6p21.3	Chromosome 6 open reading frame 10		1/6		6/8
A1364310	ESTs						6/8
AA504141	UBE2J1	6q15	Ubiquitin-conjugating enzyme E2,JI (UBC6 homolog yeast)				5/6
AA130187	WTI	11p13	Wilms tumor I	1/6			1/8
N56693	COX7B	Xq21.1	Cytochrome c oxidase subunit VIIb	5/6	1/8		
AA401441	BF	6p21.3	B-factor, properdin				1/8
AA917821	MRP530	5q11	Mitochondrial ribosomal protein S30	1/6			
A1431827	ESTs						4/8
AA935697	ESTs						3/8
A1248605	BTN3A2	6p22.1	Butyrophilin, subfamily 3, member A2				7/8
A1206970	ESTs						
AW058415	HBXIP	1p13.3	Hepatitis B virus x interacting protein	2/6			
N69107	YWHAH	22q12.3	Tyrosine 3-monooxygenase/typtophan 5-monooxygenase activation protein, eta polypeptide				1/6
AA863025	ESTs			2/6			

The ID indicates GeneBank ID, and the symbol and the cytoband information are from their source, http// source.Standford.edu. The incidence is the number of cases having log2 ratio in the range of the authors' criteria ± 0.3. ESTs are expressed sequenced tags. Clones of unknown function. Genes are listed according to order FDR values.

Table 3
Distinctive genes between types A, B (1,2), and B3

Identificatin No.	Symbol	Cytoband	Name	Type A		Type B (1,2)		Type B3	
				Gain	Loss	Gain	Loss	Gain	Loss
AA186327	SNX14	6q14-q15	Sorting nexin 14				1/14		5/8
AA287917	TNPO1	5q13.2	Karyopherin (importin) beta 2	4/6			1/14		2/8
AA442092	CTNNB1	3p21	Catenin, beta 1				1/14		1/8
AA455917	SEC22L1	1q21.2-q21.3	SEC22 vesicle trafficking protein-like 1		2/6	8/14		2/8	1/8
AA458945	RAB30	11q12-q14	RAB30, member RAS oncogene family	5/6			10/14		4/8
AA465386	DDX21		DEAD (Asp-Glu-Ala-Asp) box polypeptide 21				4/14		3/8
AA465687	RBMS1	2q23.2	Cervical cancer oncogene 4	6/6		2/14	7/14	2/8	4/8
AA478436	SMARCD2	17q23-q24	SWI/SNF-related, matrix-associated, actin department regulator of chromatin, subfamily d, member 2	6/6		3/14	6/14	1/8	2/8
AA478585	BTN3A3	6p21.3	Butyrophilin, subfamily 3, member A3	1/6					1/8
AA774608	PPPIR12B	1q32.1	Protein phosphatase 1, regulatory (inhibitor) subunit 12B					1/8	
AA931882	ESTs					3/14		5/8	
AA973568	ESTs			6/6		1/14	9/14	2/8	4/8
AA973681	ESTs			5/6			3/14		1/8
AA991868	ESTs			6/6		2/14	7/14	3/8	1/8
AA991871	FOXA1	14q12-q13	Forkhead box A1	3/6			1/14	3/8	
AI001856	ESTs		BRGI-binding protein ELD/OSA1	2/6			6/14		2/8
AI015542	TTC10	13q12.1	Probe hTg737	5/6			10/14	2/8	1/8
AI201652	ESTs			5/6			7/14	1/8	3/8
AI261862	ESTs			2/6			12/14		3/8
AI289196	MAN1A2	1p13	Mannosidase, alpha, class 1A, member 2	3/6					
AI291184	OCLN	5q13.1	Occludin	5/6		2/14	1/14		1/8
AI300984	ESTs			1/6			2/14		
AI311303	ESTs						9/14		3/8
AI335359	CI orf21	1q25	Chromosome 1 open reading frame 21					3/8	
AI337344	HSRG1	16q23.1	HSV-1 stimulation-related gene 1	6/6		1/14	8/14	3/8	2/8
AI348521	HBS1L	6q23-q24	HBS1-like				8/14		6/8
AI392929	PLU-1	1q32.1	Putative DNA/chromation binding motif					1/8	
AI401608	ESTs							2/8	

(continued on next page)

Table 3 (continued)									
Identificatin No.	Symbol	Cytoband	Name	Type A		Type B (1,2)		Type B3	
				Gain	Loss	Gain	Loss	Gain	Loss
AI492063	ESTs				2/6	1/14	3/14	5/8	
AI493835	ESTs			6/6		1/14	4/14	2/8	1/8
AI655101	XPR1	1q25.1	Xenotropic and polytropic retrovirus receptor			1/14	1/14	4/8	
AI972955	TARP	7q15-p14	T cell receptor gamma locus	1/6			7/14		
H99842	EIF5A	17p13-p12	Eukaryotic translation initiation factor 5A	2/6					

The ID indicates GeneBank ID, and the symbol and the cytoband information are from their source, http://source. standford.edu. The incidence is the number of cases having $\log_2$ratio in the range of the authors' criteria ± 0.3. ESTs are expressed sequenced tags, clones of unknown functions. Genes are listed according to order FDR values.

Data from Lee GY, Yang WI, Jeung HC, et al. Genomic-wide genetic aberrations of thymoma using cDNA microarray based comparative genomic hybridization. BMC Genomics 2007;8:305-19.

the absence of mutations in the BCL6 gene and the lack of BCL-2 and BCL-6 gene rearrangements.[28,29]

Wessendorf and colleagues performed genomic microarray on 37 PMBL specimens to further delineate the chromosomal aberrations and molecular pathways involved in the pathogenesis of PMBL.[30] In 89% of the samples, 199 chromosomal imbalances were detected. In this study, NF-κB, found to be constitutively activated in PMBL,[31] was located on chromosome 2, which demonstrated a high frequency of genomic gains using array analysis. Additionally, BCL10, a key intermediate between the T-cell receptor and NF-κB signal transduction, was found to have DNA amplification affecting chromosome 1p22. Effective gains in these two chromosomal regions suggested NF-κB activation plays a key role in PMBL pathogenesis.

Deletions in chromosomal 6p21 were detected in several PMBL specimens that corresponded to the location of the HLA (major histocomptability complex) locus.[30] Down-regulation of MHC class 2 genes has been shown to correlate with a poor prognosis in patients who have PMBL.[32] **Fig. 1** illustrates Kaplan-Meier survival data based on MHC class 2 expression in primary mediastinal B-cell lymphoma. These studies suggest that further investigation of chromosome 6p21 is needed to determine whether HLA gene deletions play a significant role in the pathogenesis of PMBL.

Activation of the janus kinases/signal transducers and activators of transcription (JAK/STAT) signal transduction pathway has been postulated to play a role in the pathogenesis of PMBL because of the high frequency of gains in chromosome 9p, the location of the JAK2 gene.[30] Impaired degradation of phosphorylated JAK2 has

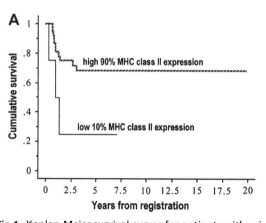
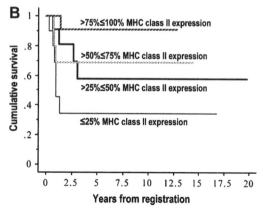

Fig. 1. Kaplan-Meier survival curves for patients with primary mediastinal large B-cell lymphoma by average MHC class 2 expression. (*A*) Survival curves based upon low 10% expressers versus the rest of the cases (*P* = .041). (*B*) Cases divided into four equal groups by MHC class 2 expression. Survival increases significantly and incrementally with increasing expression (*P* = .039).

been suggested as a mechanism for cell proliferation in PMBL.[33]

Hodgkin's Lymphoma

Hodgkin's lymphoma is characterized by rearrangement of immunoglobulin genes in most cases. Immunoglobulin gene rearrangement results in the inability to transcribe gene products or results in nonfunctional proteins.[34] Gene expression profiling demonstrated an extraordinary similar expression profile found between classic Hodgkin's lymphoma and PMBL.[34] **Fig. 2** illustrates the candidate gene expression profile of Hodgkin's lymphoma compared with PMBL and diffuse large B-cell lymphoma.

Cytogenetic analysis of classic Hodgkin's lymphoma has uncovered gains in the short arms of chromosomes 2 and 9. Gains in these chromosomes have correlated with increased gene copy numbers of the REL proto-oncogene that encodes transcriptional factors in the NF-κB family

(chromosome 2) and JAK2, which also have been hypothesized to be important in the pathogenesis of PMBL.[35] Further evidence of the role of NF-κB role in Hodgkin's lymphoma is found in one study demonstrating that NF-κB is expressed constitutively in Hodgkin's lymphoma cells. Moreover, inhibition of NF-κB activity induces apoptosis in these cells.[36]

NEUROGENIC TUMORS

Neurogenic tumors represent approximately 20% of all masses found in the mediastinum. They are classified into three groups based upon origin: nerve sheath, ganglion cell, and paraganglionic tumors.

Nerve Sheath Tumors

Most nerve sheath tumors located in the mediastinum are schwannomas and neurofibromas that are characteristically benign and slow growing.

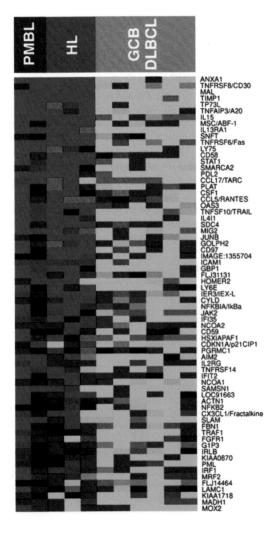

Fig. 2. Gene cluster data illustrating similar gene expression homology between primary mediastinal large B-cell lymphoma and Hodgkin's lymphoma as compared with diffuse large B-cell lymphoma. *Abbreviations:* PMBL, primary mediastinal B-cell lymphoma; HL, Hodgkin's lymphoma; GCB, germinal center B-cell; DLBCL, diffuse large B-cell lymphoma.

Neurofibromas are associated with the autosomal-dominant neurocutaneous disorder, neurofibromatosis. Normally, the NF1 gene, a tumor suppressor gene located on chromosome 17, inactivates the proto-oncogene p21-ras, thereby reducing cell proliferation.[37] In neurofibromatosis, the NF1 gene is nonfunctional, because of numerous mutational events, thereby predisposing patients who have the mutation to the development of neurofibromas throughout the body, including the posterior mediastinum. These patients have a predisposition to malignant transformation of these tumors.[38]

Ganglion Cell Tumors

Mediastinal neuroblastomas originate from the ganglion cell. Although no studies have investigated the genetic markers of neuroblastoma with regard to mediastinal disease, numerous studies have shown the importance of chromosomal aberrations in chromosome 1 in patients who have neuroblastoma.[39–41] Chromosomal loss of 1p36 and amplification of the MYCN gene have been associated with an aggressive phenotype and worse prognosis in neuroblastoma.[42]

Paraganglion Cell Tumors

Paragangliomas and pheochromocytomas are neurogenic tumors that arise from the paraganglionic cells within the thoracic cavity. No studies have investigated the genetic markers of these neurogenic tumors within the mediastinum; specifically, however, several studies have uncovered cytogenetic abnormalities and differential gene expression patterns.

Loss of heterozygosity has been reported in chromosomes 3p21[43] and 11q23[44] in paragangliomas, and on chromosomes 6q[45] and at 3p25[43] in pheochromocytomas. Recent genetic analysis has found that 25% of hereditary pheochromocytomas are caused by a germline mutation in succinate dehydrogenase B gene (SDHB), succinate dehydrogenase D gene (SDHD), Von-Hippel Lindau gene, RET gene, or the NF1 gene.[46] Furthermore, a germline mutation in the tumor suppressor gene, SDHB, is associated with a high risk of malignancy and poor prognosis in patients who have pheochromocytomas or functional paragangliomas.[46] Additionally, using quantitative polymerase chain reaction, levels of expression of hypoxic–responsive factors and angiogenic factors endothelial PAS domain protein/hypoxic inducible factor-2, hypoxic inducible factor-1, vascular endothelial growth factor (VEGF), and VEGF receptor were found to be greater in SDHD-related tumors as compared with tumors with mutations in RET or NF1.[47] This finding suggests an important link between angiogenesis and the pathogenesis of pheochromocytomas and paragangliomas.

SUMMARY

Determination of the genetic markers by the application of new genomic methodologies has provided important insight into the pathogenesis of mediastinal disease. These new techniques have enabled scientists to uncover differential gene expression patterns between subtypes of thymomas, correlate tumor marker expression with germ cell tumors, and determine a link between the NF-κB and JAK/STAT pathways with Hodgkin's and non-Hodgkin's lymphoma. Despite the progress made in the understanding of genetic markers of select mediastinal tumors, significantly more investigation is required to elucidate the molecular pathways involved in the pathogenesis of these tumors.

REFERENCES

1. Morgenthaler TI, Brown LR, Colby TV, et al. Thymoma. Mayo Clin Proc 1993;68:1110–23.
2. Detterbeck FC. Clinical value of the WHO classification system of thymoma. Ann Thorac Surg 2006;81: 2328–34.
3. Zettl A, Strobel P, Wagner K, et al. Recurrent genetic aberrations in thymoma and thymic carcinoma. Am J Pathol 2000;157:257–66.
4. Knuutila S, Bjorkqvist AM, Autio K, et al. DNA copy number amplifications in human neoplasms: review of comparative genomic hybridization studies. Am J Pathol 1998;152:1107–23.
5. Lin YW, Sheu JC, Liu LY, et al. Loss of heterozygosity at chromosome 13q in hepatocellular carcinoma: identification of three independent regions. Eur J Cancer 1999;35:1730–4.
6. Vincent A, Willcox N. The role of T-cells in the initiation of autoantibody responses in thymoma patients. Pathol Res Pract 1999;195:535–40.
7. Utada Y, Haga S, Kajiwara T, et al. Mapping of target regions of allelic loss in primary breast cancers to 1-cM intervals on genomic contigs at 6q21 and 6q25.3. Jpn J Cancer Res 2000;91:293–300.
8. Honchel R, McDonnell S, Schaid DJ, et al. Tumor necrosis factor-alpha allelic frequency and chromosome 6 allelic imbalance in patients with colorectal cancer. Cancer Res 1996;56:145–9.
9. Yeung RS, Bell DW, Testa JR, et al. The retinoblastoma-related gene, RB2, maps to human chromosome 16q12 and rat chromosome 19. Oncogene 1993;8:3465–8.

10. Berx G, Cleton-Jansen AM, Nollet F, et al. E-cadherin is a tumour/invasion suppressor gene mutated in human lobular breast cancers. EMBO J 1995;14:6107–15.

11. Zhou R, Zettl A, Strobel P, et al. Thymic epithelial tumors can develop along two different pathogenetic pathways. Am J Pathol 2001;159:1853–60.

12. Inoue M, Starostik P, Zettl A, et al. Correlating genetic aberrations with World Health Organization-defined histology and stage across the spectrum of thymomas. Cancer Res 2003;63:3708–15.

13. Shino Y, Watanabe A, Yamada Y, et al. Clinicopathologic evaluation of immunohistochemical E-cadherin expression in human gastric carcinomas. Cancer 1995;76:2193–201.

14. Sulzer MA, Leers MP, van Noord JA, et al. Reduced E-cadherin expression is associated with increased lymph node metastasis and unfavorable prognosis in nonsmall cell lung cancer. Am J Respir Crit Care Med 1998;157:1319–23.

15. Tamura S, Shiozaki H, Miyata M, et al. Decreased E-cadherin expression is associated with haematogenous recurrence and poor prognosis in patients with squamous cell carcinoma of the oesophagus. Br J Surg 1996;83:1608–14.

16. Lee GY, Yang WI, Jeung HC, et al. Genome-wide genetic aberrations of thymoma using cDNA microarray-based comparative genomic hybridization. BMC Genomics 2007;8:305.

17. Toretsky JA, Jenson J, Sun CC, et al. Translocation (11;15;19): a highly specific chromosome rearrangement associated with poorly differentiated thymic carcinoma in young patients. Am J Clin Oncol 2003;26:300–6.

18. Jain KK, Bosl GJ, Bains MS, et al. The treatment of extragonadal seminoma. J Clin Oncol 1984;2:820–7.

19. Przygodzki RM, Moran CA, Suster S, et al. Primary mediastinal and testicular seminomas: a comparison of K-ras-2 gene sequence and p53 immunoperoxidase analysis of 26 cases. Hum Pathol 1996;27:975–9.

20. Suster S, Moran CA, Dominguez-Malagon H, et al. Germ cell tumors of the mediastinum and testis: a comparative immunohistochemical study of 120 cases. Hum Pathol 1998;29:737–42.

21. Sung MT, Maclennan GT, Lopez-Beltran A, et al. Primary mediastinal seminoma: a comprehensive assessment integrated with histology, immunohistochemistry, and fluorescence in situ hybridization for chromosome 12p abnormalities in 23 cases. Am J Surg Pathol 2008;32:146–55.

22. Hiroshima K, Toyozaki T, Iyoda A, et al. Apoptosis and proliferative activity in mature and immature teratomas of the mediastinum. Cancer 2001;92:1798–806.

23. Giuliano CJ, Kerley-Hamilton JS, Bee T, et al. Retinoic acid represses a cassette of candidate pluripotency chromosome 12p genes during induced loss of human embryonal carcinoma tumorigenicity. Biochim Biophys Acta 2005;1731:48–56.

24. Looijenga LH, Oosterhuis JW. Pathogenesis of testicular germ cell tumours. Rev Reprod 1999;4:90–100.

25. Bosl GJ, Ilson DH, Rodriguez E, et al. Clinical relevance of the i(12p) marker chromosome in germ cell tumors. J Natl Cancer Inst 1994;86:349–55.

26. Copie-Bergman C, Plonquet A, Alonso MA, et al. MAL expression in lymphoid cells: further evidence for MAL as a distinct molecular marker of primary mediastinal large B-cell lymphomas. Mod Pathol 2002;15:1172–80.

27. Lazzarino M, Orlandi E, Paulli M, et al. Treatment outcome and prognostic factors for primary mediastinal (thymic) B-cell lymphoma: a multicenter study of 106 patients. J Clin Oncol 1997;15:1646–53.

28. Capello D, Vitolo U, Pasqualucci L, et al. Distribution and pattern of BCL-6 mutations throughout the spectrum of B-cell neoplasia. Blood 2000;95:651–9.

29. Tsang P, Cesarman E, Chadburn A, et al. Molecular characterization of primary mediastinal B cell lymphoma. Am J Pathol 1996;148:2017–25.

30. Wessendorf S, Barth TF, Viardot A, et al. Further delineation of chromosomal consensus regions in primary mediastinal B-cell lymphomas: an analysis of 37 tumor samples using high-resolution genomic profiling (array-CGH). Leukemia 2007;21:2463–9.

31. Feuerhake F, Kutok JL, Monti S, et al. NFkappaB activity, function, and target gene signatures in primary mediastinal large B-cell lymphoma and diffuse large B-cell lymphoma subtypes. Blood 2005;106:1392–9.

32. Roberts RA, Wright G, Rosenwald AR, et al. Loss of major histocompatibility class II gene and protein expression in primary mediastinal large B-cell lymphoma is highly coordinated and related to poor patient survival. Blood 2006;108:311–8.

33. Melzner I, Bucur AJ, Bruderlein S, et al. Biallelic mutation of SOCS-1 impairs JAK2 degradation and sustains phospho-JAK2 action in the MedB-1 mediastinal lymphoma line. Blood 2005;105:2535–42.

34. Kuppers R. Molecular biology of Hodgkin's lymphoma. Adv Cancer Res 2002;84:277–312.

35. Joos S, Granzow M, Holtgreve-Grez H, et al. Hodgkin's lymphoma cell lines are characterized by frequent aberrations on chromosomes 2p and 9p including REL and JAK2. Int J Cancer 2003;103:489–95.

36. Izban KF, Ergin M, Huang Q, et al. Characterization of NF-kappaB expression in Hodgkin's disease: inhibition of constitutively expressed NF-kappaB results in spontaneous caspase-independent apoptosis in Hodgkin and Reed-Sternberg cells. Mod Pathol 2001;14:297–310.

37. Ferner RE, Gutmann DH. International consensus statement on malignant peripheral nerve sheath

tumors in neurofibromatosis. Cancer Res 2002;62: 1573–7.

38. Strollo DC, Rosado-de-Christenson ML, Jett JR. Primary mediastinal tumors: part II. Tumors of the middle and posterior mediastinum. Chest 1997;112:1344–57.

39. Ozer E, Altungoz O, Unlu M, et al. Association of MYCN amplification and 1p deletion in neuroblastomas with high tumor vascularity. Appl Immunohistochem Mol Morphol 2007;15:181–6.

40. Scaruffi P, Parodi S, Mazzocco K, et al. Detection of MYCN amplification and chromosome 1p36 loss in neuroblastoma by cDNA microarray comparative genomic hybridization. Mol Diagn 2004;8:93–100.

41. White PS, Thompson PM, Gotoh T, et al. Definition and characterization of a region of 1p36.3 consistently deleted in neuroblastoma. Oncogene 2005; 24:2684–94.

42. Munoz J, Vendrell E, Aiza G, et al. Determination of genomic damage in neuroblastic tumors by arbitrarily primed PCR: MYCN amplification as a marker for genomic instability in neuroblastomas. Neuropathology 2006;26:165–9.

43. Vargas MP, Zhuang Z, Wang C, et al. Loss of heterozygosity on the short arm of chromosomes 1 and 3 in sporadic pheochromocytoma and extra-adrenal paraganglioma. Hum Pathol 1997;28:411–5.

44. Heutink P, van der Mey AG, Sandkuijl LA, et al. A gene subject to genomic imprinting and responsible for hereditary paragangliomas maps to chromosome 11q23-qter. Hum Mol Genet 1992;1:7–10.

45. Lemeta S, Salmenkivi K, Pylkkanen L, et al. Frequent loss of heterozygosity at 6q in pheochromocytoma. Hum Pathol 2006;37:749–54.

46. Gimenez-Roqueplo AP, Burnichon N, Amar L, et al. Recent advances in the genetics of phaeochromocytoma and functional paraganglioma. Clin Exp Pharmacol Physiol 2008;35: 376–9.

47. Gimenez-Roqueplo AP, Favier J, Rustin P, et al. The R22X mutation of the SDHD gene in hereditary paraganglioma abolishes the enzymatic activity of complex II in the mitochondrial respiratory chain and activates the hypoxia pathway. Am J Hum Genet 2001;69:1186–97.

Diagnostic Strategies for Mediastinal Tumors and Cysts

Hiroshi Date, MD

KEYWORDS

- Mediastinal tumor • Mediastinal cyst
- Diagnostic strategy • CT-guided • Ultrasound-guided

The mediastinum is an extremely important and complex part of the thorax because it contains a variety of important organs and anatomic structures. Many histologically different neoplasms and cysts that affect people of all ages arise from the multiple anatomic structures present in the mediastinum. Because this area is also the site of numerous lymph nodes, metastases secondary to lesions in other parts of the body are also frequently found. Both benign and malignant lesions are being recognized with increasing frequency, and a differential diagnosis is important whenever possible. The incidence and types of the many primary mediastinal tumors and cysts vary with the age of the patient group under consideration. In infants and children, neurogenic tumors are the most common, followed by lymphomas, foregut cysts, and benign germ cell tumors. In adults, thymic tumors are the most common surgically treated mediastinal tumors.

Treatment strategies for mediastinal tumors and cysts are quite broad, depending on the nature of the disease. This article summarizes diagnostic strategies for mediastinal tumors and cysts.

ANATOMIC COMPARTMENTS AND LOCALIZATION

Of notable significance is the division of the mediastinum into four anatomic compartments, because specific lesions characteristically arise in certain locations. The mediastinum is demarcated by the thoracic inlet superiorly, the diaphragm inferiorly, mediastinal pleura laterally, the sternum anteriorly, and the vertebral column posteriorly. The notion of anatomic compartments is of practical value whenever one is deriving a differential diagnosis for a given mediastinal mass. A plane extending from the lower manubrium to the fourth thoracic vertebra separates the superior from the inferior mediastinum. The inferior compartment is further subdivided by the pericardium into anterior, middle, and posterior compartments (**Fig. 1**). The superior mediastinum contains the upper third of the thoracic esophagus, the great vessels, the upper trachea, the superior vena cava, the upper pole of the thymus gland, and the peritracheal and paratracheal lymph nodes. This is the area into which a thyroid mass, such as a retrosternal thyroid goiter, can descend. The contents of the anterior mediastinum are mediastinal fat and the body and lower poles of the thymus gland. The middle mediastinum contains the pericardium, heart, aorta, carina and main bronchi, and bronchial lymph nodes. The esophagus, descending aorta, the thoracic duct, and the sympathetic chain are located in the posterior mediastinum.

The tumors and cysts most commonly occurring in each of the four mediastinal compartments are depicted in **Fig. 2**. There are rare exceptions with each lesion, such as the occasional neurogenic tumor arising in the anterior mediastinum or an ectopic thyroid tumor located in the posterior mediastinum.

SIGNS AND SYMPTOMS

Although a number of mediastinal lesions are found by a routine chest radiographic examination in an asymptomatic patient, approximately

Department of Thoracic Surgery, Kyoto University Graduate School of Medicine, 54 Shogoin Kawahara-cho, Sakyo-ku, Kyoto 606-8507, Japan
E-mail address: hdate@kuhp.kyoto-u.ac.jp

Thorac Surg Clin 19 (2009) 29–35
doi:10.1016/j.thorsurg.2008.09.001
1547-4127/08/$ – see front matter © 2009 Elsevier Inc. All rights reserved.

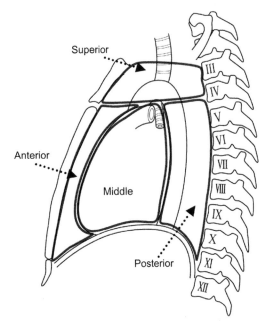

Fig. 1. Four anatomic compartments of the mediastinum.

two-thirds of patients have specific symptoms. A variety of presenting signs and symptoms may be present in patients depending on whether the lesion is benign or malignant, its size, its location, the presence or absence of infection, the elaboration of specific endocrine or other biochemical products, and the presence of associated systemic disease states.

The most common presenting complaints include chest pain, cough, and dyspnea. When malignant disease is present, signs and symptoms of direct anatomic invasion or compression—such as hoarseness, Horner's syndrome, diaphragmatic paralysis, chylothorax, and superior vena caval syndrome (**Fig. 3**)—are generally associated with a poor prognosis. Symptoms and signs from compression of vital structures by benign lesions are uncommon because most normal, mobile, mediastinal structures can conform to distortion from pressure.

Systemic symptoms are rare, but typically are caused by the release of excess hormones and antibodies. Ectopic thyroid tumors may be associated with thyrotoxicosis. Parathyroid adenomas, occasionally found in the mediastinum, are associated with the clinical and laboratory findings of hyperparathyroidism. Thymic carcinoid tumors may be associated with Cushing's syndrome. Gynecomastia is present in over half of the patients with mediastinal choriocarcinoma and is believed to result from β-human chorionic gonadotropin (hCG) production. Hypertension occurs in association with mediastinal pheochromocytomas and ganglioneurinomas, and diarrhea may also be associated with these lesions. Myasthenia gravis is known to occur more frequently in the presence of thymoma. Thymomas have also been reported in association with pure red blood cell aplasia, hypogammaglobulinemia, and other autoimmune diseases.

EXAMINATION METHODS

When a mediastinal lesion is recognized on standard radiographs of the chest, the diagnostic possibilities can be narrowed to a reasonable number by considering the patient's age, the location of the mass, and the associated symptoms and signs present. At first, a careful evaluation of the history,

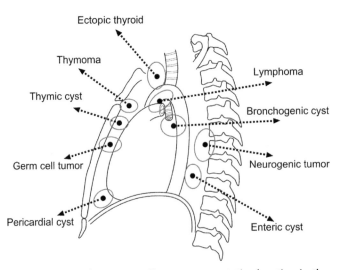

Fig. 2. Common mediastinal tumors and cysts according to representative location in the mediastinum.

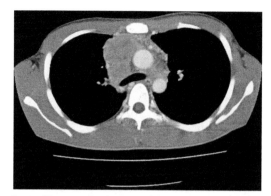

Fig. 3. CT scan of a 24-year-old man presenting with facial edema reveals a solid bulky mass of the anterior mediastinum that completely occludes superior vena cava. Diagnosis of thymoma was established by percutaneous CT-guided needle biopsy.

signs, and symptoms is valuable. Various imaging modalities are currently available and provide excellent depiction of the mediastinal lesions. The main imaging modalities used are chest radiography, CT, MRI, and positron emission tomography (PET).

CT is routinely indicated when a mediastinal lesion is detected by chest radiography. The rapid acquisition of the entire thorax during a single breath-hold minimizes motion artifacts and allows optimal vascular contrast enhancement.[1] It allows a reliable evaluation of the mediastinal anatomy and the relationship of the lesions with adjacent structures. CT is a sensitive method of distinguishing between fatty, vascular, cystic, and soft tissue masses. However, the differentiation of a cyst and a solid tumor is not always accurate.[2]

MRI may supply additional useful information in separating mediastinal tumors from vessels and bronchi, especially when the use of contrast material is contraindicated. MRI is more accurate than CT in assessing tumor invasion to the great vessels, heart, and chest wall, and in distinguishing a cyst from a solid tumor.[3,4] T1-weighted images are most valuable in anatomic assessment, whereas T2-weighted images are most valuable in tissue characterization. A cyst has homogeneous high-signal intensity on the T2-wighted image and can be distinguished from a solid tumor.

PET using fluorine-18 fluorodeoxyglucose (FDG) has emerged as a diagnostic tool for staging several types of neoplasms. Fusion of FDG-PET with CT images (PET/CT) further increases the diagnostic accuracy by depicting more precisely the anatomic site of uptake and avoiding misinterpretation of normal hypermetabolic area as disease. FDG-PET is useful in differentiating thymoma from hyperplasia in myasthenia gravis,[5] and may be useful for predicting the grade of malignancy in thymic epithelial tumors.[6]

Radioisotope scanning has been of specific aid in establishing a definitive diagnosis for ectopic thyroid and parathyroid tumors.

Biochemical makers and elevated hormone levels are present in patients with various mediastinal tumors. Infants and children with a paravertebral mass should be evaluated for excessive norepinephrine and epinephrine production. This increased production is present in association with most neuroblastomas and ganglioneuroblastomas. Young adult men with an anterior mediastinal mass should have determinations of levels of α-fetoprotein and β-hCG. Either one or both are elevated in the presence of a nonseminomatous germ cell tumor. Antiacetylcholine receptor antibodies should be measured in patients with thymoma because occult myasthenia gravis may be found. Serum-soluble interleukin-2 receptors may be elevated in the presence of mediastinal lymphoma. Hypokalemia, high-serum cortisol, and adrenocorticotropic hormone (ACTH) levels are seen in some patients with thymic carcinoid tumors that produce an ectopic secretion of ACTH.

METHODS FOR PATHOLOGIC DIAGNOSIS

The precise nature of a lesion in the mediastinum, as elsewhere, cannot be determined without pathologic diagnosis. It is often required to confirm a presumed diagnosis and to select the optimal treatment modality. A variety of biopsy techniques for obtaining tissue from the mediastinum have been described, including ultrasound (US)-guided endoscopic biopsy, percutaneous image-guided needle biopsy, parasternal anterior mediastinotomy, cervical mediastinoscopy, video-assisted thoracoscopic surgery, and open surgical procedures.

Percutaneous US-Guided Needle Biopsy

Ultrasonography is an effective modality for guidance of percutaneous biopsy. Compared with CT, US-guided biopsy offers a number of advantages, including bedside approach, lower cost, lack of radiation exposure, and real-time monitoring.[7] With real-time monitoring by means of US guidance, the tip of the biopsy-needle can be monitored throughout the procedure. Another great advantage of US-guided biopsy is that it can approach the lesion from any direction. This advantage allows biopsy of an upper mediastinal lesion via a supraclavicular approach (**Fig. 4**). CT-guided biopsy of this region is usually hindered by surrounding bony structures at an axial plane. On the other hand, the greatest limitation of US-guided biopsy is that its clinical application for thoracic lesions is generally confined to anterior- or

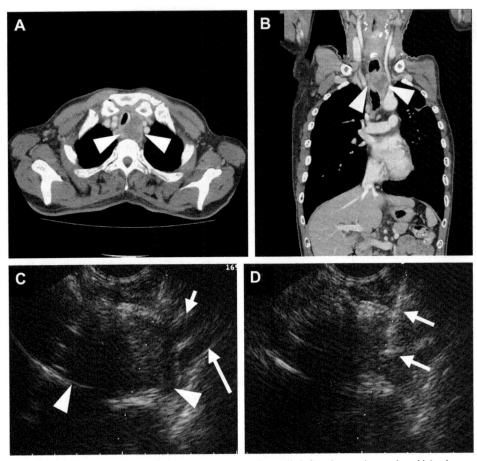

Fig. 4. (*A*) Contrast enhanced CT of a 64-year-old man reveals an ill-defined mass (*arrowheads*) in the upper mediastinum. The mass is located posterior to the bony structures, including sternum, first rib, and proximal clavicle. (*B*) Multiplanar reformation image of contrast-enhanced CT demonstrates an upper mediastinal tumor (*arrowheads*) medial to the left common carotid artery. (*C*) Ultrasonograph from left supraclavicular approach shows the upper mediastinal mass (*arrowheads*). Left subclavian vein (*short arrow*) and artery (*long arrow*) can be recognized laterally to the puncture guide (*dotted line*). The interval between the dots measures 1 cm. (*D*) Ultrasonograph of the mass at the moment of tissue sampling. The needle of high ecogenecity (*arrows*) intervene into the mass. Subsequent pathologic examination yielded carcinoma of unknown primary.

posterior-mediastinal tumors that are in contact with the chest wall.

Patients are examined with real-time, linear, convex, and sector US units with 3.5- MHz and 5.0-MHz transducers. The US units equipped with Doppler US may be preferable, as Doppler US can be used to detect vessels and blood flow that should be avoided from the biopsy root. After confirming the biopsy root, the US probe is equipped with a sterile puncture transducer with a guiding channel. A commonly used biopsy needle is an 18-gauge biopsy gun (Bard Max Core; CR Bard Inc., Tempe, AZ), which consists of an outer cannula and an inner obturator with a 20-mm specimen notch at the tip. When the puncture probe reaches the lesion, the cutting needle is passed through the guiding channel and introduced into the margin of the lesion. The inner obturator is automatically fired by pushing the firing button, and is rapidly followed by the outer cannula to cut off the tumor tissue in the specimen notch. Subsequently, the entire unit is withdrawn. If the lesion is less than 20 mm to 22 mm in diameter, the tip of the needle should be placed at least 20 mm away from the posterior margin of the lesion. To reduce the false-negative rate, having a cytologist present during biopsy has been advocated.[8]

Percutaneous CT-Guided Needle Biopsy

This procedure is performed percutaneously under CT-fluoroscopic guidance.[9] The instrument the author uses is a coaxial biopsy system consisting of a 19-gauge introducer needle (Co-Axial

Introducer Needle; Medical Device Technologies, Gainesville, FL) and a 20-gauge core biopsy needle (Super-Core II Biopsy Instrument; Medical Device Technologies). Before the procedure, CT images are obtained for targeting the lesion. The needle path is determined, avoiding interlobular fissures, visible bronchi, and relatively large vessels. The needle path may be through the lung (**Fig. 5**), a route that cannot be used in US-guided biopsy. After the administration of local anesthesia, the introducer needle is advanced along the determined path until its tip is in front of the lesion. The internal stylet is removed and the biopsy needle is immediately replaced. The stylet of the biopsy needle is advanced into the lesion. A specimen is obtained by pressing the plunger, and the biopsy needle is removed followed by immediate replacement by the stylet of the introducer needle. Acquisition of a specimen is repeated until the specimens obtained are considered adequate for histologic evaluation. The introducer needle is removed to finish the procedure and chest CT images are obtained to evaluate procedural complications.

Pneumothorax (8%–61%) is the most commonly encountered complication after US-guided or CT-guided needle biopsy, followed by hemoptysis (1.6%–3%).

US-Guided Endoscopic Biopsy

Endobronchial ultrasound (EBUS), first introduced during the early 1990s, has emerged as a new diagnostic tool that allows visualization beyond the airway.[10] Because of the development of miniaturized radial probes with flexible catheters having a balloon at the tip (**Fig. 6**), bronchoscopists can

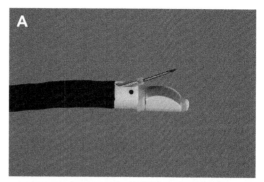

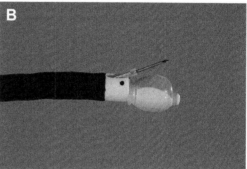

Fig. 6. (*A*) Tip of the ultrasound puncture bronchoscope (CP-EBUS, Olympus XBF- UC260F-OL8) with the linear curved array ultrasonic transducer. (*B*) The balloon attached to the top of the bronchoscope is inflated with normal saline and a dedicated 22-gauge aspiration needle is protruded from the biopsy channel.

perform real-time EBUS-guided transbronchial needle aspiration (EBUS-TBNA). Although EBUS-TBNA is mainly used for lymph node staging in lung cancer, it can also be used for tissue diagnosis for middle mediastinal lesions. A 22-gauge needle is passed through the airway wall and inserted into the lesion under real-time ultrasound control. Esophageal US-guided fine-needle aspiration needle biopsy is sometimes indicated for the posterior- and inferior-mediastinal lesions.

EBUS-TBNA is minimally invasive and can be performed quite safely under local anesthesia. The disadvantages are that the tissue sample is small, the procedure is time-consuming and technically demanding, and it requires expensive tools. It is for these reasons that this procedure can be performed only in some centers.

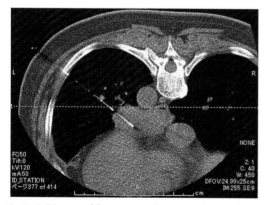

Fig. 5. A 54-year-old woman with a posterior mediastinal tumor. CT fluoroscopic image during the procedure with the patient in the pone position shows a biopsy needle introduced into the mediastinal tumor though the lung. Diagnosis of leiomyoma was established pathologically.

Parasternal Anterior Mediastinotomy

When needle biopsy has failed, many surgeons prefer Chamberlain's approach:[11] an open biopsy using a parasternal anterior mediastinotomy. The patient is placed under general anesthesia in a supine position. Local anesthesia is occasionally used. A 3-cm to 4-cm transverse parasternal skin incision is made at the desired intercostal space, depending on the location of the tumor. Great care should be taken to stay lateral to the internal mammary vessels. Under direct visualization between the ribs and using biopsy forceps, an adequately sized specimen can be obtained from an anterior mediastinal tumor. Para-aortic lesions and masses arising from the aortopulmonary window can be reached by inserting a mediastinoscope through the parasternal incision.

Mediastinoscopy

Conventional mediastinoscopy and recently developed videomediastinoscopy are generally used for evaluating the mediastinal lymph nodes in patients with carcinoma of the lung. These techniques are also useful for the diagnosis of mediastinal lesions located in the pretracheal, paratracheal, and subcarinal spaces.[12] Under general anesthesia, a small transverse incision is made 2 cm above the sternal notch. The pretracheal fascia is incised and a tunnel created by gentle finger dissection along the anterior and lateral walls of the trachea in to the mediastinum. The mediastinoscope is then introduced and advanced further by means of blunt instrument dissection to extend the mediastinal tunnel. Great care should be taken to avoid vascular injury and left-recurrent nerve palsy. An adequately sized tissue sample can be obtained using biopsy forceps.

Video-Assisted Thoracoscopic Surgery

Video-assisted thoracoscopic surgery (VATS) has been widely used for various types of thoracic surgery. Under general anesthesia, the patient is intubated with a double-lumen endotracheal tube and placed in a lateral decubitus position. With the lung collapsed, the entire thoracic cavity is visible. VATS is a valuable procedure, especially in cases of lesions with difficult access that require direct vision, such as tumors close to great vessels or the heart.[13,14] The disadvantage of VATS biopsy for mediastinal tumor is possible tumor seeding to the thoracic cavity by opening the pleura.

Decision-Making

One can make a reasonable preoperative diagnosis for each lesion by considering the age of the patient, location, the presence or absence of symptoms and signs, the association of a specific systemic disease, radiographic findings, and biochemical markers. The decision about how to manage a mediastinal tumor could be made by observation, surgical resection, chemotherapy, radiotherapy, or multimodality therapy, depending on the nature of the disease.

Since the introduction of VATS, the threshold for surgical resection of the lesion has been lowered. In most patients with cystic lesions or probable benign solid tumors, such as neurogenic tumors in adults, VATS extirpation of the lesion is recommended without biopsy, being both diagnostic and therapeutic simultaneously. When radiographs show typical signs of benign germ cell tumors, mature teratomas, or early stage thymomas, the author recommends open or VATS resection without biopsy.

It is much more difficult to make a precise diagnosis for poorly demarcated tumors in the anterior or middle mediastinum. Thymomas, thymic carcinomas, seminomas, nonseminomatous germ cell tumors, and lymphomas are quite similar in radiographic appearance but are quite different in treatment strategy. Therefore, pathologic diagnosis is required to select the optimal treatment modality.

Several techniques and approaches have been previously described and are available to obtain specimens of mediastinal tumors. The choice of technique depends on the location of the lesion, clinical factors such as the age and the condition of the patient, and the availability of special techniques with the required expert and the necessary equipment. In general, percutaneous biopsy is the first diagnostic choice because it can be done under local anesthesia.

REFERENCES

1. Storto ML, Ciccotosto C, Patea RL, et al. Spiral CT of the mediastinum: optimization of contrast medium use. Eur J Radiol 1994;18(Suppl 1):S83–7.
2. Mendelson DS, Rose JS, Efremidis SC, et al. Bronchogenic cysts with high CT numbers. Am J Roentgenol 1983;140(3):463–5.
3. Muller NL. Computed tomography and magnetic resonance imaging: past, present and future. Eur Respir J Suppl 2002;35:3s–12s.
4. Jeung MY, Gasser B, Gangi A, et al. Imaging of cystic masses of the mediastinum. Radiographics 2002; 22(Spec No):S79–93.
5. El-Bawab H, Al-Sugair AA, Rafay M, et al. Role of fluorine-18 fluorodeoxyglucose positron emission tomography in thymic pathology. Eur J Cardiothorac Surg 2007;31(4):731–6.
6. Endo M, Nakagawa K, Ohde Y, et al. Utility of (18)FDG-PET for differentiating the grade of malignancy in thymic epithelial tumors. Lung Cancer 2008;61(3):350–5.
7. Wernecke K, Vassallo P, Peters PE, et al. Mediastinal tumors: biopsy under US guidance. Radiology 1989; 172(2):473–6.

8. Austin JH, Cohen MB. Value of having a cytopathologist present during percutaneous fine-needle aspiration biopsy of lung: report of 55 cancer patients and metaanalysis of the literature. Am J Roentgenol 1993;160(1):175–7.

9. Güllüoǎlu MG, Kiliçaslan Z, Toker A, et al. The diagnostic value of image guided percutaneous fine needle aspiration biopsy in equivocal mediastinal masses. Langenbecks Arch Surg 2006;391(1):222–7.

10. Yasufuku K, Nakajima T, Chiyo M, et al. Endobronchial ultrasonography: current status and future directions. J Thorac Oncol 2007;2(10):970–9.

11. Olak J. Parasternal mediastinotomy. Chest Surg Clin N Am 1996;6(1):31–40.

12. Carlens E. Mediastinoscopy: a method for inspection and tissue biopsy in the superior mediastinum. Dis Chest 1956;36(10):343–52.

13. Yim AP, Lee TW, Izzat MB, et al. Place of video-thoracoscopy in thoracic surgical practice. World J Surg 2001;25(2):157–61.

14. Rendina EA, Venuta F, De Giacomo T, et al. Comparative merits of thoracoscopy, mediastinoscopy, and mediastinotomy for mediastinal biopsy. Ann Thorac Surg 1994;57(4):992–5.

Infections of the Mediastinum

Kalliopi A. Athanassiadi, MD, PhD

KEYWORDS

- Mediastinal infection • Acute mediastinitis
- Chronic mediastinitis
- Esophageal perforation • Poststernotomy complication

Mediastinal infection (ie, mediastinitis) has four possible sources: (1) direct contamination, (2) hematogenous or lymphatic spread, (3) extension of infection from the neck or retroperitoneum, and (4) extension from the lung, pleura, or chest wall. The organs and tissues involved determine the manifestations and approach to treatment of these infections. In the preantibiotic era, most cases of mediastinitis resulted from extension of infections from adjacent structures (primarily head and neck infections), though they were occasionally due to extension of pulmonary and pleural infections. Today, the most common cause of mediastinitis is direct invasion of the mediastinum after surgical intervention. According to the definition of mediastinitis established by The Centers for Disease Control and Prevention in the United States,[1] diagnosis of mediastinitis requires at least one of the following:

An organism from culture isolated of mediastinal tissue or fluid

Evidence of mediastinitis seen during operation

One of the following conditions: chest pain, sternal instability or fever (>38°C) in combination with either (1) purulent discharge from the mediastinum or an organism isolated from the blood culture or (2) cultural or mediastinal drainage

Mediastinitis may be either acute or chronic. Both are usually infectious in etiology. Acute mediastinitis is due to a bacterial infection and chronic mediastinitis is usually related to a granulomatous infection, such as histoplasmosis.

ACUTE MEDIASTINITIS

Acute mediastinitis is a serious infection involving the connective mediastinal tissue that fills the interpleural spaces and surrounds the mediastinal organs.[2] The majority of acute mediastinal infections result from esophageal perforation (posterior mediastinitis) or infection following a transsternal cardiac procedure (anterior mediastinitis) or even penetrating trauma. Occasionally, acute mediastinitis results from odontogenic, peritonsillar infections that cause oropharyngeal abscesses with severe cervical infection spreading along to the fascial planes into the mediastinum.[3,4] Acute mediastinitis may also result from iatrogenic oropharyngeal perforation, cervical trauma, epiglottitis, parotitis, sinusitis, sternoclavicular joint infection, and illicit intravenous drug administration. Furthermore, any surgical procedure on the neck, including lymph node biopsy, thyroidectomy, tracheostomy, and mediastinoscopy, could cause subsequent mediastinitis, but such a development is very rare. The fascial planes in the neck that are continuous with those in the mediastinum facilitate extension of the infection from the neck. The retrovisceral, pretracheal, and carotid sheath spaces allow direct extension downward. Gravity, respiration, and negative intrathoracic pressure are believed to forward intrathoracic spread.[5]

This is described as descending necrotizing mediastinitis. Estrera and colleagues,[6] in accurately defining the diagnosis, include the following criteria:

Clinical manifestation of severe oropharyngeal infection

Department of Thoracic Surgery, General Hospital of Piraeus, Athens-Greece, 34A Konstantinoupoleosstr., Holargos, 15562 Athens, Greece
E-mail address: kallatha@otenet.gr

Thorac Surg Clin 19 (2009) 37–45
doi:10.1016/j.thorsurg.2008.09.012
1547-4127/08/$ – see front matter © 2009 Elsevier Inc. All rights reserved.

Demonstration of characteristic radiological features of mediastinitis

Documentation of necrotizing mediastinitis at operation or postmortem examination or both

Establishment of relationship between oropharyngeal infection and development of necrotizing mediastinal process

Spread of infection from the retroperitoneum or subphrenic areas to the mediastinum has been described for many years and remains an important though infrequent cause of acute mediastinitis.[6]

Microbiology

Infections resulting from esophageal perforations or secondary to spread from odontogenic infections might be caused by gram-negative aerobic, as well as anaerobic, organisms. The most common anaerobic organisms are anaerobic *Streptococcus* and *Bacteroides* spp.[5] Usually, in acute mediastinitis, infections are polymicrobial. Particular attention should be given to the usual oral pharyngeal flora, including *Candida* and *Aspergillus* in the deteriorating or debilitated patient.[7] Mediastinitis secondary to rib or vertebral osteomyelitis is extremely rare, but has been described in cases of tuberculosis or fungal infections.[4]

Clinical Features

Patients with acute mediastinitis usually present with acute onset of symptoms, including fever and leucocytosis, chest pain, dysphagia, and respiratory distress. The cervical infection, when present, is easily recognized, since the patient complains of edema, neck pain, dysphagia, and odynophagia.[8] Dysphagia is also characteristic of esophageal perforation while respiratory distress indicates pleural involvement, either pleural effusion or pneumothorax, especially in adults.

Radiological Findings

Chest radiographs may demonstrate diffuse mediastinal widening and findings associated with mediastinal abscess, including gas bubbles or a fluid level.[9] Pneumomediastinum and pneumothorax are usually associated with esophageal perforation and are not often seen in other cases of mediastinitis. Pleural or pericardial effusion may also be present. In cases of esophageal perforation, esophagograms with meglumine diatrizoate (Gastrografin) are used to confirm the diagnosis, although it is reported that such esophagograms can be false negative in 10% to 25% of cases.[10] Barium is avoided because of the possible risk of barium-induced mediastinal inflammation (**Fig. 1**).

CT scan is the diagnostic tool of choice because it is more sensitive than other diagnostic tools in determining the degree of mediastinal involvement. CT may reveal the presence and the extent of mediastinal fluid collection and the presence of extraluminal gas, pericardial and pleural effusions, and soft tissue edema[9] (**Fig. 2**). Additionally, a CT scan can also evaluate the relationship of the fluid collections to the adjacent thoracic and extrathoracic structures.[9] In that context, evaluation of the peritoneum and retroperitoneum is imperative to exclude the presence of infection. Cervical CT is imperative in cases of descending necrotizing mediastinitis because it helps detect the cause of infection[11] (**Fig. 3**).

Additionally, a CT scan can play a role in guiding drainage procedures.[12] Marty-Ane and colleagues[5] and Freeman and colleagues[13] stressed the importance of CT scanning also in the perioperative period in assessing the surgical drainage and the timing for a possible reoperation. Cervicothoracic CT imaging is usually repeated after any operative drainage or debridement and with any deterioration of the patient's clinical condition. The evaluation might be completed by abdominal CT imaging when the patient's clinical condition fails to improve or deteriorates in the presence of a normal cervicothoracic CT scan or if the patient's symptoms are consistent with an intra-abdominal infection.[13]

Treatment

Treatment should be directed toward the primary pathology and the clinical presentation. Intravenous administration of a broad-spectrum

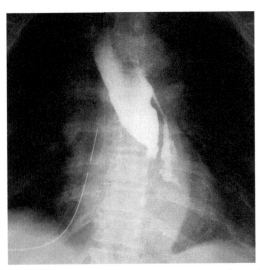

Fig. 1. Esophagogram demonstrating an esophageal perforation, and a drained pleural effusion.

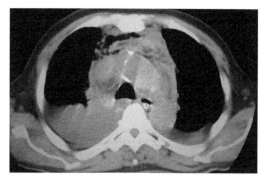

Fig. 2. Thoracic CT scan showing an anterior acute mediastinitis associated with upper mediastinal tissue edema, distortion of tissue planes, and bilateral effusions.

antibiotic, such as piperacillin-tazobactam, should be initiated and modified as culture and sensitivity results become available. Correction of hypovolemia secondary to sepsis and third-space losses into the mediastinum with appropriate intravenous fluids should be undertaken.[4]

Surgical drainage remains the gold standard, but the surgical approach to the mediastinum and particularly the optimal form of mediastinal drainage remains controversial and ranges from cervical drainage alone to cervical drainage along with routine thoracotomy or thoracoscopy.[3–6,8,14,15] Knowledge of the cervical fascial planes is essential to understand the pathways, symptoms, and complications of cervical infections.[3–5]

All procedures should be performed by a multidisciplinary team comprising a head and neck surgeon and a thoracic surgeon. In cases where an odontogenic abscess is the cause, synchronous treatment by maxillofacial surgeons is essential.

The consensus view seems to be that an aggressive cervical approach (cervicotomy) should be undertaken. The neck is often approached either through a longitudinal incision along the anterior border of the sternocleidomastoid muscle or through a transverse collar bilateral incision or both. The involved cervical spaces are opened, drained, and debrided of necrotic tissue and the cervical wound is left open. The wound should heal by second intention (**Fig. 4**). The upper anterior mediastinum can be entered transcervically through the pretracheal space and opened by blunt finger dissection to the level of tracheal bifurcation, while the upper posterior is entered by extending the dissection of the retropharyngeal space downward.[5,6,8]

When the mediastinal infection expands below the carina or the T4 vertebra, a transthoracic approach should be considered;[5,6] the procedure includes opening the mediastinal pleura on a longitudinal axis, debridement of the mediastinum, and complete excision of necrotic tissue. If necessary, along with the drainage of the pleural cavity, a decortication or even insertion of chest tubes for mediastinopleural irrigation might take place. Debridement of necrotic tissue is essential.

In a review by Wheatley and colleagues,[16] 12 of 43 patients (28%) underwent only transcervical drainage, while 20 of 43 (46%) initially managed through cervicotomy required subsequent thoracotomy, since the infection was extended to the lower mediastinum.

For optimal drainage and debridement of the chest, the literature mentions various approaches, such as the subxiphoid approach, clamshell incision, and median sternotomy, while some investigators recently reported thoracoscopic drainage or debridement with or without minithoracotomy.[5,6,17–22]

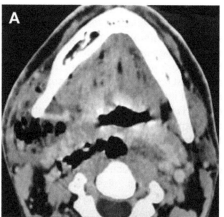

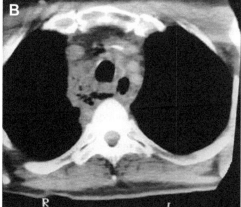

Fig. 3. CT scan of a patient with acute posterior mediastinitis due to cervical abscess. (*A*) Cervical CT scan demonstrates the cervical abscess. (*B*) The infection progresses through the posterior mediastinum.

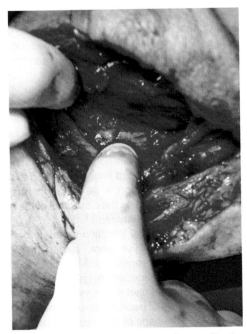

Fig. 4. Drainage of the upper posterior mediastinum through a cervical incision.

Corsten and colleagues[23] reported the advantages of posterolateral thoracotomy in addition to cervical drainage alone by showing a significant difference in mortality in patients who received neck and thoracic drainage (19%) compared with neck drainage alone (47%). Casanova and colleagues[17] achieved complete thoracic drainage through a median sternotomy in two patients. Ris and colleagues[19] performed a clamshell incision in three cases because of the possible difficulty of gaining access to the posterobasal compartments of the chest cavity through sternotomy, especially on the left side. According to Ris and colleagues,[19] the approach through a clamshell incision offers an excellent exposure for a complete one-stage operation, including bilateral decortication and debridement of the mediastinum along with pericardiectomy, if necessary, avoiding at the same time potential complications, such as sternal dehiscence and osteomyelitis. Each of the above-mentioned methods has advantages and disadvantages.

Video-assisted thoracic surgery can be of great help. When employed early enough, video-assisted thoracic surgery enables easy exploration and drainage in selective cases.[21,24] Furthermore, video-assisted mediastinoscopy for the drainage of mediastinal abscesses above the carina has been mentioned in the literature and may be considered as an option.[25]

At the present time, posterolateral thoracotomy remains the best approach. It exposes the prevertebral and paraesophageal spaces and allows access to the ipsilateral mediastinum and the pericardium in cases where the infection extends below the tracheal bifurcation. Also, unlike sternotomy or clamshell incision, posterolateral thoracotomy carries no risk of sternal osteomyelitis. The choice of site depends on the site of the collection. Tracheostomy is often necessary but should be performed selectively.

Unfortunately, high mortality rates (25%–50%) are reported, despite the introduction of modern antimicrobial therapy and CT imaging.[12,19,21,26] Delay in diagnosis and delayed or inappropriate drainage of the mediastinum are the main causes for the high mortality. The delay between onset of primary infection and hospitalization varied in different series from 5 to 22 days and represented an important factor contributing to the mortality reported.[2,27] As infection spreads along deep cervical planes into the mediastinum, widespread cellulitis, necrosis, abscess formation, and sepsis may occur.[7] Complications include adult respiratory distress syndrome, acute renal failure, pneumonia, and chylothorax.

Freeman and colleagues[13] published an interesting algorithm for patients with deep-space infections. This algorithm calls for the initial use of broad-spectrum antibiotics along with the use of a contrast-enhanced cervicothoracic CT imaging to recognize early descending necrotizing mediastinitis. When infection is present, neck and thoracic drainage followed by debridement is essential. Repetition of CT is useful within 48 to 72 hours to identify any progression of the infection. In cases of progression, further surgical therapy is necessary.

Treatment of acute mediastinitis due to esophageal perforation with direct spillage of the mediastinum with gastric contents should be separately discussed. Negative thoracic pressure by respiratory efforts and positive gastric pressure promotes further drainage into the mediastinum and pleural space.[28] Conservative treatment consists of parenteral or enteral nutrition, antibiotic administration, nasogastric suctioning, administration of histamine-2 receptor blockers, and pleural drainage.[29] At an early stage of esophageal rupture, surgical intervention is indicated. The method of choice is primary repair of the laceration reinforced by a flap of a well-vascularized tissue and mediastinal debridement. Resection procedures with or without reconstruction should be done only in exceptional cases, such as in cases involving underlying esophageal disease or malignancy.[29,30] There is still a continuing discussion about the most appropriate treatment in cases of delay. Some series[31] suggest esophagectomy, while others insist on primary repair regardless of the time of presentation.[29,32–34] In cases with advanced mediastinitis and necrosis of the esophageal wall, different techniques have been advocated, such as esophageal exclusion or extirpation with cervical esophagostomy and gastrostomy.[31,34]

Covered self-expanding metal stents have proven useful in palliating malignant esophageal perforations and fistulas. Complications reported include migration; adverse effects of the endoprothesis on normal esophageal tissues, including pressure-induced ischemia, ulceration, and perforation and reactive stenoses at the ends of the endoprothesis; bleeding or injury on removal; and unsuccessful retrieval.[35,36] More experience is needed for assessment of the potential role and complications of stent insertion. However, in cases of delayed diagnosis or patient's poor general condition, the placement of a self-expandable stent might effectively control mediastinal spillage.

It is suggested that treatment should be individualized in each patient because the disease process is not uniform in acute mediastinitis, which still remains a life-threatening infection. Therapy will improve with a better understanding of the natural history of the disease and its anatomic spread, along with CT surveillance, promotes improvements in therapy.

POSTSTERNOTOMY MEDIASTINITIS

Poststernotomy mediastinitis in cardiac surgery represents an infrequent but serious problem because subsequent sepsis seeding to the heart, suture lines, and prosthetic conduits or valves can be life-threatening.[37–42] Risk factors involved in cases of poststernotomy mediastinitis are multiple and include obesity, diabetes mellitus, chronic obstructive pulmonary disease, coexistence of peripheral vascular disease, and bilateral use of internal mammary artery.[43–45] Recent progress in cardiac surgery has meant that an increasing number of elderly and immunosupressed patients with multiple risk factors are treated surgically. Therefore, despite in-hospital infection control and antibiotic treatment, the incidence of mediastinitis has remained constant over the years. While some papers fail to report mortality, in the majority that do, the mortality ranges from 16.5% to 47%.[46] Death may be caused by generalized sepsis, endocarditis, fatal hemorrhage, or secondary multiple organ dysfunction, as well as nosocomial superinfections. Moreover, deep sternal infections leave physical, mental, and cosmetic scars, and often cause prolonged hospitalization.[47]

Microbiology

In cases of poststernotomy mediastinitis, the spectrum is very broad. The infection includes gram-negative and gram-positive bacteria as well as fungi.[48] *Staphylococcus aureus* found in the skin flora seems to be the most common species.[43,49] Aerobic streptococci, coagulase-negative staphylococci, *Pseudomonas aeruginosa* and *Enterococcus* have been also isolated. Sternal puncture is a rapid and safe method to confirm the diagnosis.[50]

Treatment

An effective treatment is required to avoid high morbidity and mortality in these patients. In 1963, Schuhmacher and Mandelbaum[37] introduced antibiotic irrigation, debridement, and reclosure of the sternum. In 1976, Lee and colleagues[39] described sternal excision with wide debridement of bone cartilage and transposition of the well-vascularized omentum with primary closure, while Jurkiewicz and colleagues[40] used a muscle flap. Banic and colleagues[51] reported the use of latissimus dorsi as a free myocutaneous flap in cases of extensive sternectomy.

Today the most commonly used muscle for sternal reconstruction is the pectoralis major followed by rectus abdominis and greater omentum flaps or a combination of flaps.[51–54] As Pairolero[42] suggested, the surgeon's first choice, when different muscles have been tried without success, is to obliterate the mediastinal space and use the omentum, the so-called "policeman of the abdomen," as a back-up flap. It is well known that the omental flap easily fills the cavity after complete or partial sternal excision and obliterates the dead space. It contains large numbers of immunologically active cells, which seem to be responsible for the omentum's high anti-infective activity. Its extensive vascularization, as well as its neovascularization potential, increases the blood supply, leading to higher concentration of antibiotics at the infection site. By absorbing wound secretion, it eliminates substrates for bacterial growth.

Finally, the omentum can be harvested rapidly, resulting to a short operation time. The procedure does not require specific knowledge and can be performed by any surgeon. By contrast, mobilizing and rotating the pectoralis muscles centrally on the thoracoacromial vessels[54] and performing direct skin closure or using a myocutaneous latissimus dorsi flap is a time-consuming operation that should be performed by a specialist thoracic or plastic surgeon. Some investigators[55–57] advocate the laparoscopic harvesting of the omental flap as a substitute for the traditional laparotomy.

In 1995, Calvat and colleagues[47] followed by Trouillet and colleagues[58] proposed closed drainage by using redon catheters for local treatment. For both, results were good, but neither classified mediastinal infection according to the system proposed by El Oakley and Wright.[41]

Recently, vacuum-assisted closure has come to represent an emerging and safe alternative modality for wound healing in patients with deep sternal infection, although its effectiveness in mediastinitis types III and IV has not been proven.[59,60] Vacuum-assisted closure is based on the application of local negative pressure on the wound. Polyurethane foam with an open-pore structure of 400 to 600 μm is placed in the wound. One end of a tube is connected to the foam and the other to the vacuum source. The wound is covered by a drape so that an airtight system is created. A continuous or intermittent negative pressure is applied. It allows open drainage with stabilization of the chest and isolation of the wound and promotes tissue granulation. Because these systems are portable, patients can be mobilized earlier and get physiotherapy so that further complications are minimized.

In conclusion, no consensus has emerged about which treatment for poststernotomy mediastinitis is the most effective. Surgical revision with open dressings or closed irrigation followed by sternal rewiring or secondary healing might be accompanied by a mortality rate as high as 45%.[41,61–66] Open dressings produce thoracic instability requiring longer intubation and mechanical ventilation in the intensive care unit. Prolonged immobilization also causes additional complications, such as pneumonia, thrombosis, and muscular weakness. Therefore, reconstruction with vascularized muscle flaps or omentum is advised in cases of mediastinitis type III and IV, although it creates an even greater surgical challenge if reoperation is needed. Topical negative pressure therapy[49] is a good alternative, especially in cases of type I and II.

CHRONIC MEDIASTINITIS

Chronic mediastinitis might be produced by an acute mediastinitis or may be secondary to granulomatous processes, including such infections as histoplasmosis, syphilis, tuberculosis, coccidiomycosis, and, less commonly, noninfectious granulomatous processes, such as sarcoidosis.[3,4,9,67,68] Sclerosing mediastinitis due to *Histoplasma capsulatum*, which is common in North America, is usually associated with other sites of fibrosis, such as the retroperitoneum, the thyroid gland, the orbit, and the cecum.[4,9] Chronic mediastinitis has been also associated with immunologic abnormalities, such as lupus erythematosus, rheumatoid arthritis, Raynaud's phenomenon, and such drugs as methysergide.[3,4,67] Finally, foreign bodies that were not removed might result in chronic mediastinitis.

Clinical Manifestations

Patients with chronic mediastinitis are usually asymptomatic. If symptoms occur, they usually arise secondary to compression or obstruction of major airways and vascular structures (superior vena cava, pulmonary arteries and veins).[63,67,68,69] These symptoms are nonspecific and include cough, dyspnea, wheezing, chest pain, dysphagia, and hemoptysis. The clinical picture in the progressive disease can mimic a malignant process, which has to be excluded.

Radiologic Findings

On chest radiograph, mediastinal fibrosis may present as diffuse widening. In cases where the mediastinitis is due to granulomatous disease, calcification is identified within enlarged and mediastinal lymph nodes. CT scan is far more sensitive than chest radiographs in detecting lymph nodes, fibrosis, and calcification, while contrast-enhanced CT scan is the diagnostic tool of choice in detecting vascular compression. Lung abnormalities might also be identified in patients with chronic mediastinitis due to sarcoidosis, tuberculosis, or fungal infection.[9] For differential diagnosis between benign and malignant disease, MRI plays an important role because, in benign mediastinal fibrosis, only low-intensity signals on both T1 and T2 images are present. Also, MRI enables good evaluation of vascular patency.[9]

Treatment

No treatment has been widely accepted. Surgical intervention is only justified to establish a diagnosis. Bronchoscopy, mediastinoscopy, or mediastinotomy is performed and specimens should be examined in the cytology or pathology and microbiology departments.[67] Biopsy should be done cautiously because there is a high tendency for bleeding as extensive fibrosis is present. Only as a palliative measure should patients be submitted to resection of enlarged compressive granulomatous lymph nodes. The procedure might lessen the likelihood of subsequent progressive fibrosis.[67] Stenting of vascular structures or excision and reconstruction with prosthetic grafts or even tracheal resection are mentioned in the literature.[63,69]

The treatment of chronic mediastinitis is relatively troublesome. Antimicrobial and chemotherapeutic agents have been tried, but they are seldom successful.[4,67] Excision of involved tissues is often necessary to alleviate symptoms of compression. However, surgical intervention is seldom considered and is used only in a supportive role, usually late in the course of the disease.

REFERENCES

1. Mangram AJ, Horan TC, Pearson ML, et al. Guideline for prevention of surgical site infection, 1999. Centers for Disease Control and Prevention (CDC) Hospital Infection Control Practices Advisory Committee. Am J Infect Control 1999;27:97–132.
2. Papalia E, Rena O, Oliaro A, et al. Descending necrotizing mediastinitis: surgical management. Eur J Cardiothorac Surg 2001;20:739–42.
3. Fry WA, Shields TW. Acute and chronic mediastinal infections. In: Shields TW, editor. Mediastinal surgery. Philadelphia: Lea & Febiger; 1991. p. 101–8.
4. Ewing HP, Hardy ID. The Mediastinum. In: Baue AE, Geha AS, Hammond GI, et al, editors. 5th edition, Glenn's thoracic & cardiovascular surgery, vol. I. Norwalk (CT): Appleton & Lang; 1991. p. 584–7.
5. Marty-Ane Ch-H, Berthet J-P, Alric P, et al. Management of descending necrotizing mediastinitis: an aggressive treatment for an aggressive disease. Ann Thorac Surg 1999;68:212–7.
6. Estrera AS, Lanay MJ, Grisham JM, et al. Descending necrotizing mediastinitis. Surg Gynecol Obstet 1983;157:545–52.
7. Kiernan PD, Hernandez A, Byrne WD, et al. Descending cervical mediastinitis. Ann Thorac Surg 1998;65:1483–8.
8. Van Natta TL, Lannetoni MD, et al. Acute necrotizing mediastinitis. In: Patterson GA, Cooper JD, Deslauriers J, et al, editors. 3rd edition, Pearson's thoracic & esophageal surgery, vol. I. Philadelphia: Churchill Livingstone; 2008. p. 1521–8.
9. Boiselle PhM. Diffuse mediastinal abnormalities. In: McLoud ThC, editor. Thoracic radiology, the requisites. St Louis (MO): Mosby; 1998. p. 464–7.
10. Goldstein LA, Thompson WR. Esophageal perforations: a 15-year experience. Am J Surg 1992;143:495–503.
11. Brunelli A, Sabbatini A, Catalini G, et al. Descending necrotizing mediastinitis: surgical drainage and tracheostomy. Arch Otolaryngol Head Neck Surg 1996;122:1326–9.
12. Gobien RP, Stanley JH, Gobien BS, et al. Percutaneous catheter aspiration and drainage of suspected mediastinal abscesses. Radiology 1984;151:69–71.
13. Freeman RK, Vallieres E, Verrier ED, et al. Descending necrotizing mediastinitis: an analysis of the effects of serial surgical debridement on patient mortality. J Thorac Cardiovasc Surg 2000;119(2):260–7.
14. Pearse HE. Mediastinitis following cervical suppuration. Ann Surg 1938;108:588–91.
15. Marty-Ane CH, Alauzen M, Alric P, et al. Descending necrotizing mediastinitis: advantage of mediastinal drainage with thoracotomy. J Thorac Cardiovasc Surg 1994;107:55–61.
16. Wheatley MJ, Kirsch S, Ggo O, et al. Descending necrotizing mediastinitis: Transcervical drainage is not enough. Ann Thorac Surg 1990;49:780–4.
17. Casanova J, Bastos P, Barreiros F, et al. Descending necrotizing mediastinitis—successful treatment using a radical approach. Eur J Cardiothorac Surg 1997;12:494–6.
18. Gorlitzer M, Grabenwoeger M, Meinhart J, et al. Descending necrotizing mediastinitis treated with rapid sternotomy followed by vacuum-assisted therapy. Ann Thorac Surg 2007;83:393–6.
19. Ris HB, Banij A, Furrer M, et al. Descending necrotizing mediastinitis: surgical treatment via clamshell approach. Ann Thorac Surg 1996;62:1650–4.
20. Isowa N, Yamada T, Kijima T, et al. Successful thoracoscopic debridement of descending necrotizing mediastinitis. Ann Thorac Surg 2004;77:1834–7.
21. Roberts JR, Smythe WR, Weber RW, et al. Thoracoscopic management of descending necrotizing mediastinitis. Chest 1997;112:850–4.
22. Nagayasu T, Sh Akamine, Tadayuki O, et al. Thoracoscopic drainage with wound edge protector for decending necrotizing mediastinitis. Inter Cardiovasc Thorac Surg 2003;2:58–60.
23. Corsten MJ, Shamji FM, Odell PF. Optimal management of descending necrotizing mediastinitis. Thorax 1997;52:702–8.
24. Min H-K, Choi YC, Shim YM, et al. Descending necrotizing mediastinitis: a minimally invasive approach using video-assisted thoracoscopic surgery. Ann Thorac Surg 2004;77:306–10.
25. Shimizu K, Otani Y, Nakano T, et al. Successful video-assisted mediastinoscopic drainage of descending necrotizing mediastinitis. Ann Thorac Surg 2006;81:2279–81.
26. Sancho LMM, Minamoto H, Fernadez A, et al. Descending necrotizing mediastinitis: a retrospective surgical experience. Eur J Cardiothorac Surg 1999;16:200–5.
27. El-Ebrahim KE. Descending necrotizing mediastinitis: a case report and review of the literature. Eur J Cardiothorac Surg 1995;9:161–2.
28. Lemke T, Jagminas L. Spontaneous esophageal rupture: a frequently missed diagnosis. Am Surg 1999;65:449–52.
29. Eroglu A, Kurkcuoglu IC, Karaoglanoglu N, et al. Esophageal perforation: the importance of early diagnosis and primary repair. Dis Esophagus 2004;17:91–4.

30. Kiernan PD, Sheridan MJ, Hettrick V, et al. Thoracic esophageal perforation: one surgeon's experience. Dis esoph 2006;19:24–30.

31. Salo JA, Seppala KMY, Pitkaranta PP, et al. Spontaneous rupture and functional status of the esophagus. Surgery 1992;112(5):897–900.

32. Port JL, Kent MS, Korst RJ, et al. Thoracic esophageal perforations: a decade of experience. Ann Thorac Surg 2003;75:1071–4.

33. Jones WG II, Ginsberg RJ. Esophageal perforation: a continuing challenge. Ann Thorac Surg 1992;53: 534–43.

34. Kotsis L, Agocs L, Kovacs J. Transhiatal closure of right-sided rupture after a left pneumonectomy. Ann Thorac Surg 1997;63:246–7.

35. Yuasa N, Hattori T, Kobayashi Y, et al. Treatment of spontaneous esophageal rupture with a covered self-expanding metal stent. Gastrointest Endosc 1999;49(6):777–80.

36. Koch S, Weber A, Fein F, et al. Prothese oesophagiennes expansives extirpables dans le traitement des perforations non tumorales del'oesophage. Gastroenterol Clin Biol 2005;29:735–9.

37. Schuhmacher HB, Mandelbaum I. Continuous antibiotic irrigation in the treatment of infection. Arch Surg 1968;86:54–7.

38. Bryant LR, Spencer FC, Trinkle JK. Treatment of median sternotomy infection by mediastinal irrigation with an antibiotic solution. Ann Surg 1969;169: 914–20.

39. Lee AB, Schimert G, Shaktin S, et al. Total excision of the sternum and thoracic pedicle transposition of the greater omentum: useful strategies in managing severe mediastinal infection following open heart surgery. Surgery 1976;80:433–6.

40. Jurkiewicz MJ, Bostwick J, Hester TR, et al. Infected median sternotomy wound. Successful treatment with muscle flaps. Ann Surg 1980;191:738–44.

41. El Oakley RM, Wright JE. Postoperative mediastinitis: classification and management. Ann Thorac Surg 1996;61:1030–6.

42. Pairolero PC, Arnold PG. Management of infected median sternotomy wounds. Ann Thorac Surg 1986;42:1–2.

43. Borger MA, Rao V, Weisel RD, et al. Deep sternal wound infection: risk factors and outcomes. Ann Thorac Surg 1998;65:1050–6.

44. The Parisian Mediastinitis Study Group. Risk factors for deep sternal wound infection after sternotomy: a prospective, multicenter study. J Thorac Cardiovasc Surg 1996;111:1200–7.

45. Antunes PE, Bemando JE, Eugenio L, et al. Mediastinitis after aorto-coronary bypass surgery. Eur J Cardiothorac Surg 1997;12:443–9.

46. De Feo M, Renzulli A, Ismeno G, et al. Variables predicting adverse outcome in patients with deep sternal wound infection. Ann Thorac Surg 2001;71:324–31.

47. Calvat S, Trouillet J, Nataf P, et al. Closed drainage using Redon catheters for local treatment of poststernotomy mediastinitis. Ann Thorac Surg 1996; 61:195–201.

48. Sjoegren J, Malmsjö M, Gustafsson R, et al. Poststernotomy mediastinitis: a review of conventional surgical treatments, vacuum-assisted closure therapy and presentation of the Lund University Hospital mediastinitis algorithm. Eur J Cardiothorac Surg 2006;30:898–905.

49. Segers P, De Jong AP, Kloek JJ, et al. Poststernotomy mediastinitis: comparison of 2 treatment modalities. Inter Cardiovasc Thorac Surg 2005;4:555–60.

50. Benlolo S, Mateo J, Raskine L, et al. Sternal puncture allows an early diagnosis of poststernotomy mediastinitis. J Thorac Cardiovasc Surg 2003;125(3): 611–7.

51. Banic A, Ris HB, Emi D, et al. Free latissimus dorsi flap for chest wall repair after complete resection of infected sternum. Ann Thorac Surg 1995;60: 1028–32.

52. Schroeyers P, Wellens F, Degrieck I, et al. Aggressive primary treatment for poststernotomy acute mediastinitis: our experience with omental and muscle flaps surgery. Eur J Cardiothorac Surg 2001;20: 743–6.

53. El Gamel A, Yonan NA, Hassan R, et al. Treatment of mediastinitis: early modified Robicsek closure and pectoralis major advancement flaps. Ann Thorac Surg 1998;65:41–7.

54. Francel TJ, Kouchoukos NT. A rational approach to wound difficulties after sternotomy: reconstruction and long-term results. Ann Thorac Surg 2001;72: 1419–29.

55. Domene CE, Volpe P, Onari P, et al. Omental flap obtained by laparoscopic surgery for reconstruction of the chest wall. Surg Laparosc Endosc 1998;8(3): 215–8.

56. Avital S, Rosin D, Brasesco O, et al. Laparoscopic mobilization of an omental flap for reconstruction of an infected sternotomy wound. Ann Plast Surg 2002;49(3):307–11.

57. Puma E, Fedeli C, Ottavi P, et al. Laparoscopic omental flap for the treatment of major sternal wound infection after cardiac surgery. J Thorac Cardiovasc Surg 2003;126(6):1998–2002.

58. Trouillet J-L, Vuagnat A, Combes A, et al. Acute poststernotomy mediastinitis managed with debridement and closed-drainage aspiration: factors associated with death in the intensive care unit. J Thorac Cardiovasc Surg 2005;129(30):518–24.

59. Gustafsson RI, Sjoegren J, Ingemansson R. Deep sternal wound infection: a sternal-sparing technique with vacuum-assisted closure therapy. Ann Thorac Surg 2003;76:2048–53.

60. Fuchs U, Zittermann A, Stuettgen B, et al. Clinical outcome of patients with deep sternal wound infection

managed by vacuum-assisted closure compared to conventional therapy with open packing: a retrospective analysis. Ann Thorac Surg 2005;79:526–31.

61. Sarr MG, Gott VL, Townsend TR. Mediastinal infection after cardiac surgery. Ann Thorac Surg 1984; 38:415–23.

62. Luciani N, Lapenna E, De Bonis M, et al. Mediastinitis following graft replacement of the ascending aorta: conservative approach by omental transposition. Eur J Cardiothorac Surg 2001;20:418–20.

63. Bays S, Rajakaruma Ch, Sheffield Ed, et al. Fibrosing mediastinitis as a cause of superior vena cava syndrome. Eur J Cardiothorac Surg 2004;26:453–5.

64. Karra R, McDermont L, Connelly S, et al. Risk factors for 1-year mortality after postoperative mediastinitis. J Thorac Cardiovasc Surg 2006;132(3):537–43.

65. Yoshida K, Ohshima H, Murakami F, et al. Omental transfer as a method of preventing residual persistent subcutaneous infection after mediastinitis. Ann Thorac Surg 1997;63:858–9.

66. Raman J, Song DH, Bolotin G, et al. Sternal closure with titanium plate fixation—a paradigm shift of preventing mediastinitis. Inter Cardiovasc Thorac Surg 2006;5:336–9.

67. Urschel HC Jr, Patel AN, Razzuk MA, et al. Chronic mediastinitis. In: Patterson GA, Cooper JD, Deslauriers J, editors. 3rd edition, Pearson's thoracic & esophageal surgery, vol. I. Philadelphia: Churchill Livingstone; 2008. p. 1529–36.

68. Mathisen DJ, Grillo HC. Clinical manifestation of mediastinal fibrosis and histoplasmosis. Ann Thorac Surg 1992;54:1053–8.

69. Kalweit G, Huwer H, Straub U, et al. Mediastinal compression syndromes due to idiopathic fibrosing mediastinitis—report of 3 cases and review of the literature. Thorac Cardiovasc Surg 1996;44(2):105–9.

Mediastinal Tumors and Cysts in the Pediatric Population

Cameron D. Wright, MD

KEYWORDS

• Pediatric • Mediastinal tumor • Mediastinal cyst

Mediastinal masses in children have many similarities to those in adults; the mediastinal compartment where the mass is predominately located remains the beginning point. Unlike in adults, large masses can cause life-threatening airway compression because of the combination of the relatively smaller size and greater compressability of the pediatric airway. In addition, the incidence of malignancy among the various compartment locations varies between adults and children. However, similar to adults, most mediastinal tumors and cysts require excision. The mediastinal compartment from which the mass primarily rises helps to narrow the differential diagnosis, similar to adult patients (**Tables 1–3**). However, the relative proportion of the various entities is different between children and adults. This relative difference is best exemplified in a recent report of 806 mediastinal masses from a single Japanese institution that treated both adult and pediatric populations (**Table 4**).[1] The prevalence of malignancy was 37% in the children and 47% in the adults (thymomas stage II and above were considered malignant). Symptoms were present in 53% of the children and 49% of the adults overall. The prevalence of symptoms in malignant tumors was 73% in the children and 75% in the adults. Thymic tumors are most common in adults and neurogenic tumors are most common in children (**Table 5**). The chest radiograph and chest CT usually provide enough information, in combination with the age and clinical history, to provide a focused differential diagnosis of the pediatric mediastinal mass. Consultation with a pediatric radiologist often provides invaluable help in rapidly arriving at the correct diagnosis. Franco, Mody, and Meza recently reviewed the radiologic evaluation of pediatric mediastinal masses.[2]

ANTERIOR MEDIASTINAL MASSES
The Normal Pediatric Thymus

The normal pediatric thymus is relatively larger than in adults and it is important in the development of the child's immune system. It normally weighs about 15 g at birth and 35 g at puberty, at which time it involutes and is gradually replaced with fat. The size of the thymus is correlated to the weight of the infant. The generous thymus in infancy is sometimes mistaken for true pathology causing superior anterior mediastinal widening (**Figs. 1** and **2**). On CT, the thymus has the same density as muscle and enhances with contrast injection (**Fig. 3**). With MR imaging, the thymus has a homogeneous intensity; if there is significant inhomogeneity, a pathologic process should be suspected. T-1 images are a little brighter than muscle and T-2 images are much brighter than muscle. The normal pediatric thymus has increased uptake of fluorodeoxyglucose (FDG) and thus, PET scans are of limited use in evaluating the pediatric thymus.

Ectopic Thymus

Ectopic thymus can be found anywhere in the neck or chest but is usually found along the pathway of descent from the angle of the mandible to the mediastinum. Most commonly, ectopic thymus is found in the right paratracheal location (**Fig. 4**).[3]

Thymic Hyperplasia

Thymic hyperplasia is a rare disorder whereby the thymus, for unknown reasons, is markedly enlarged without disruption of the normal architecture. It is not a neoplastic process, but the enlarged thymus can compress vital structures

Blake 1570, Division of Thoracic Surgery, Massachusetts General Hospital, 55 Fruit St, Boston, MA, USA
E-mail address: cdwright@partners.org

Thorac Surg Clin 19 (2009) 47–61
doi:10.1016/j.thorsurg.2008.09.014
1547-4127/08/$ – see front matter © 2009 Elsevier Inc. All rights reserved.

Table 1
Pediatric anterior mediastinal masses

Thymus
Normal thymus
Thymic hyperplasia
Thymic cyst
Thymoma

Lymphadenapathy
Infectious
Lymphoma

Tumors
Germ cell tumors
Teratomas
Seminomas
Nonseminomatous germ cell tumors
Hemangiomas
Lymphangiomas

Table 3
Pediatric posterior mediastinal masses

Ganglion cell tumors
Neuroblastoma
Ganglioneuroma
Ganglioeuroblastoma

Other nerve tumors
Schwannoma
Neurofibroma
Paraganglioma
Meningocele

Rarely pleural metastases may be seen. The tumors enhance with contrast. Complete resection is the mainstay of obtaining a diagnosis and cure. The approach is usually by mediansternotomy. Staging and prognosis are identical to adult thymomas.[5] Adjuvant radiation is typically not given for completely resected Masaoka stage II and III thymomas because of the late complications of adjuvant mediastinal radiation in the child.

such as the lung (**Fig. 5**).[4] Thymic hyperplasia is associated with Grave's disease, myasthenia gravis, and chemotherapy.

Thymic Cysts

Thymic cysts can present in the neck, span the neck and mediastinum, or present entirely in the mediastinum. They are usually unilocular but can be multiloculated. They may compress vital structures and thus are removed for diagnosis and treatment.[6]

Thymomas

Thymomas are rare in children, representing only 1%–4% of all mediastinal masses in children. As in adults, they may be asymptomatic or present with compressive symptoms. CT imaging demonstrates a soft tissue mass usually in the anterior mediastinum with projection into one of the pleural spaces (**Fig. 6**). Usually the margins are smooth, but with invasive thymomas they can be irregular. Occasional areas of calcification may be seen.

Lymphoma

Among malignant tumors in children, lymphomas are relatively common. Non-Hodgkin's lymphomas predominate while Hodgkin's lymphoma occurs in about one third of cases.[7] The mediastinum is frequently involved with lymphomas in children. There is usually an inhomogeneous mediastinal mass with lymphadenopathy

Table 2
Pediatric middle mediastinal masses

Lymphadenapathy
Lymphoma
Infection

Tumors
Nerve tumors
Hemangioma

Cysts
Bronchogenic cyst
Esophageal duplication cyst
Pericardial cyst

Table 4
Mediastinal tumor location in children and adults

Location	Adults	Children
Anterior	68%	36%
Middle	18%	12%
Posterior	14%	52%

Data from Takeda S, Miyoshi S, Akinori A et al. Clinical spectrum of primary mediastinal tumors: A comparison of adult and pediatric populations at a single Japanese institution. J Surg Oncol 2003;83:24–30.

Table 5
Mediastinal tumors and cysts in adults and children

TumorType	Adults	Children
Thymic	36%	4%
Germ cell tumors	16%	19%
Cysts	14%	8%
Lymphomas	12%	13%
Neurogenic tumors	11%	46%

Data from Takeda S, Miyoshi S, Akinori A et al. Clinical spectrum of primary mediastinal tumors: A comparison of adult and pediatric populations at a single Japanese institution. J Surg Oncol 2003;83:24–30.

(**Figs. 7** and **8**). There are often areas of necrosis and compression of vital structures. Non-Hodgkin's lymphoma presents in younger children while Hodgkin's disease usually presents in the adolescent or young adult. Often the diagnosis can be made by biopsy of a cervical lymph node, but direct biopsy of the mediastinal mass is occasionally necessary. The treatment is with chemotherapy.

GERM CELL TUMORS
Teratomas

Teratomas are the most common mediastinal germ cell tumor and are composed of all three germinal layers. They are usually in the anterior mediastinum closely associated with the thymus and

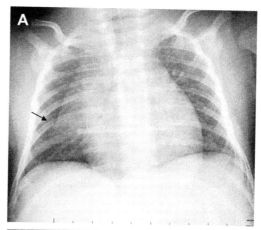

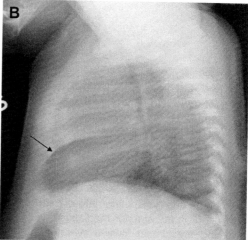

Fig. 2. Thymic sail sign. Four month-old infant presenting with shortness of breath. Frontal (*A*) and lateral (*B*) radiographs of the chest demonstrate a normal thymus with the sail sign representing flattening of the lower margin of the gland abutting the minor fissure (*arrows*). (*From* Franco A, Mody NS, Meza MP. Imaging evaluation of pediatric mediastinal masses. Radiol Clin N Am 2005;43:328; with permission.)

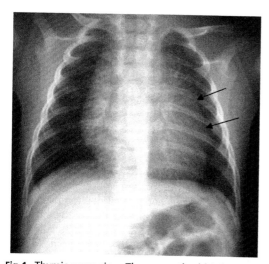

Fig. 1. Thymic wave sign. Three-month-old infant presenting with vomiting. Undulations of the left lobe of the normal thymus (*arrows*) are caused by the adjacent costal cartilage. (*From* Franco A, Mody NS, Meza MP. Imaging evaluation of pediatric mediastinal masses. Radiol Clin N Am 2005;43:327; with permission.)

present with a large mass. They may also protrude into the neck from the mediastinum. They appear benign and encapsulated and they are frequently cystic (**Fig. 9**). They are often inhomogeneous with areas of cystic change, solid tissue, and areas of calcification. They contain mature ectodermal elements such as hair, skin and neuroglial elements. Other tissues may be present including, bone, cartilage, teeth, muscle, fat and endocrine tissue. Excision confirms the diagnosis and is the treatment of choice. Teratomas may contain immature elements that act aggressively and provide yet another reason to remove all teratomas.[8,9]

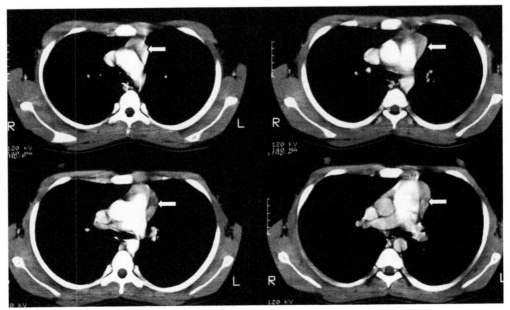

Fig. 3. CT appearance of normal thymus. A 12-year-old boy presenting with chest pain at an outside hospital. The CT was considered suspicious for lymphoma. A series of axial images from an intravenous contrast-enhanced chest CT demonstrate homogeneous enhancement of prominent but normal left thymic lobe (*arrows*). (*From* Franco A, Mody NS, Meza MP. Imaging evaluation of pediatric mediastinal masses. Radiol Clin N Am 2005;43:328; with permission.)

Malignant Germ Cell Tumors

Seminomas and nonseminomatous germ cell tumors occur in the anterior mediastinum in young boys and are almost always symptomatic with compressive symptoms. Seminomas are marker negative, while nonseminomatous tumors present with elevation of the markers beta HCG or alpha fetoprotein. Seminomas are usually large invasive homogeneous masses that rarely calcify. Nonseminomatous tumors are large invasive inhomogeneous tumors with areas of necrosis and hemorrhage (**Fig. 10**). Seminomas require fine needle aspiration for diagnosis, while nonseminomatous tumors can be diagnosed by tumor marker elevation alone in association with the clinical and radiologic scenario. The treatment is with cisplatin-based chemotherapy. Residual masses in the nonseminomatous tumors require resection. About 50% of patients with nonseminomatous tumors are cured, while almost all seminomas are cured.[10,11]

Lymphangiomas

Cystic lymphangiomas, also known as cystic hygromas, are uni- or mulilocular cysts filled with clear or straw colored fluid lined by epithelium derived from lymphatic vessels. There is a prediliction for these to occur in the neck, but they can also span from the neck to the mediastinum or be solely in the mediastinum. Most present in infancy and 90% present within the first 2 years of life. Isolated medastinal cystic lymphagiomas are usually asymptomatic.[12,13] Ultrasound is helpful in superficial cervical lesions, while CT and MR are helpful in mediastinal and deep lesions. Resection is recommended upon diagnosis. Although resection should be complete, radical en-bloc resection of vital structures is not prudent. Cyst injection with sclerosing agents (OK-432, 22.5% glucose) is considered for extensive cystic lymphangiomas when surgery is not possible.

Hemangiomas

Hemangiomas are proliferative lesions characterized by increased endothelial cell turnover. They typically grow rapidly after birth and then involute over time. They can be in any mediastinal compartment. They are usually asymptomatic and well circumscribed on imaging. They may compromise adjacent structures by direct extension or by compression. Asymptomatic lesions are typically observed for involution. Medical therapy with steroids, interferon, propanolol, and embolization are done for symptomatic lesions. Resection is rarely performed.[14,15]

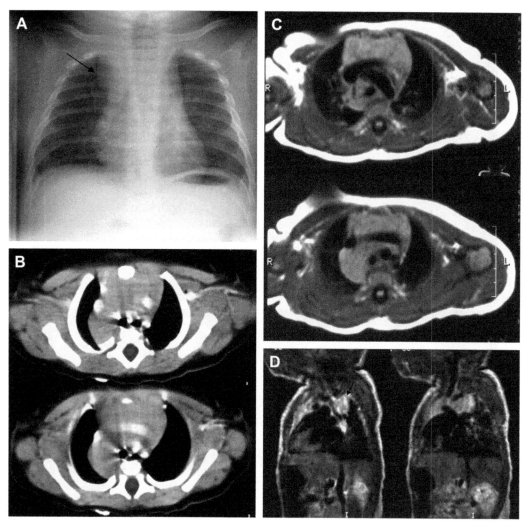

Fig. 4. Right paratrachealetopic thymus. Three-month-old infant presenting with fever. There is an abnormal contour (*arrows*) along the right upper mediastinal margin on frontal radiograph (*A*). A series of contrast-enhanced axial CT images of the chest (*B*) confirm the posterior location of tissue with attenuation identical to the normally positioned thymus within the anterior mediastinum. Axial (*C*) and sagittal oblique (*D*) contrast-enhanced T1-weighted MR images also demonstrate continuity and identical signal intensity of the ectopic thymus with the anterior thymus (*arrow*). (*From* Franco A, Mody NS, Meza MP. Imaging evaluation of pediatric mediastinal masses. Radiol Clin N Am 2005;43:331; with permission.)

Middle Mediastinal Masses

Foregut (duplication) cysts are benign cystic mediastinal lesions that are derived from the primitive foregut that normally gives origin to the tracheobronchial tree and the esophagus.

Bronchogenic Cysts

Bronchogenic cysts are the most common cystic lesion of the mediastinum. The cysts are lined with respiratory tract ciliated columnar epithelium or cuboidal epithelium containing mucus glands. The accumulation of mucus causes gradual enlargement of bronchogenic cysts. The cyst wall is composed of fibroelastic tissue, smooth muscle, and cartilage. They may occur anywhere along the tracheobronchial tree but are most common around the carina and right hilum. Rarely, they are found in the neck, lung, pleura, pericardium or subdiaphragmatic. They are not associated with other congenital anomalies. Infants present with airway obstructive symptoms, and older children present with infectious or inflammatory complications. CT typically demonstrates a spherical non-enhancing mass of variable attenuation with sharp borders (**Fig. 11**). Rarely an air-fluid level is present if there is patent communication with the airway.

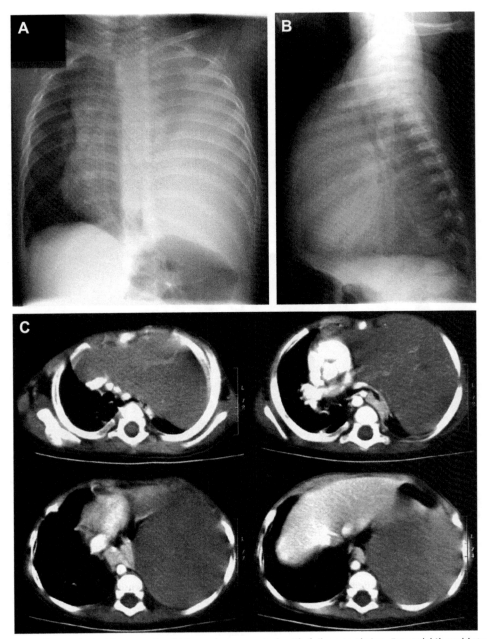

Fig. 5. Thymic hyperplasia. Nine-month-old boy who presented with failure to thrive. Frontal (*A*) and lateral (*B*) radiographs reveal a large, left-sided mass with shift of the mediastinum to the right and loss of volume of the left lung. (*C*) Representative images from an intravenous contrast-enhanced CT examination reveal a large, homogenous mass in the anterior mediastinum displacing the heart and great vessels posteriorly and to the right. The left lung is severely compressed. (*From* Franco A, Mody NS, Meza MP. Imaging evaluation of pediatric mediastinal masses. Radiol Clin N Am 2005;43:331; with permission.)

The density of the cyst is higher than water because mucus fills the cyst (typically 30–120 Hounsfield units). Cysts are typically excised for diagnosis and treatment when discovered. Infectious complications are thought to be frequent enough to warrant routine excision. If a cyst is actively infected, then surgery should, in general, be delayed for a course of antibiotic treatment. The approach is either by video-assisted thoracic surgery (VATS) or lateral thoracotomy depending on the complexity of the cyst and the experience of the surgeon.[16–18]

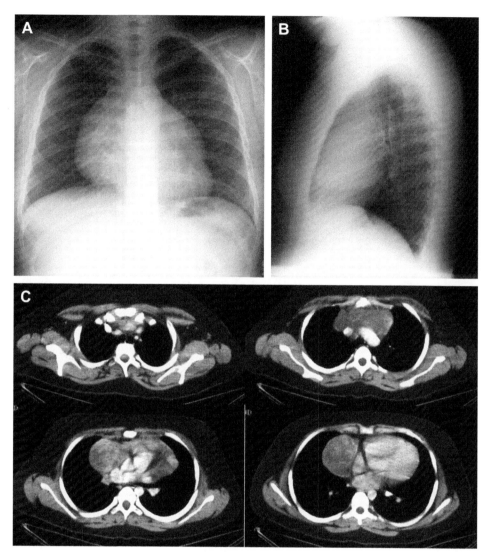

Fig. 6. Thymoma. An otherwise healthy 8-year-old boy presenting with chest pain. Frontal (*A*) and lateral (*B*) chest radiographs demonstrate an anterior mediastinal mass. (*C*) A series of axial intravenous contrast-enhanced images of the chest show a large, lobulated anterior mediastinal mass with irregular enhancement. (*From* Franco A, Mody NS, Meza MP. Imaging evaluation of pediatric mediastinal masses. Radiol Clin N Am 2005;43:332; with permission.)

Esophageal Duplication Cysts

Esophageal duplication cysts are rare cystic lesions of the mediastinum and are usually located along the idle or lower esophagus. They are about one tenth as common as bronchogenic cysts in most series. Rarely, more distal enterogenous duplications may extend through the diaphragmatic hiatus and simulate an esophageal duplication cyst. The cyst can be tubular or spherical and cysts are typically intimate with the wall of the esophagus. Rarely, the duplication cyst may extend into the spinal canal, which is known as a neuroenteric cyst. Most of these cysts are asymptomatic. They rarely present with airway compression, dysphagia, or peptic ulceration from ectopic gastric mucosa in the cyst. Patients with an esophageal duplication cyst may have a second duplication cyst elsewhere along the alimentary tract. They are also associated with a variety of skeletal abnormalities, including spina bifida, hemivertebra, vertebral fusion, and spinal extension of the duplication cyst. CT demonstrates a smooth-edged cystic lesion without calcification with homogeneous lower attenuation (15–30 Hounsfield units) (**Fig. 12**). Resection is indicated for all

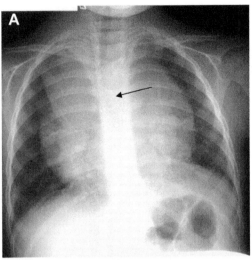

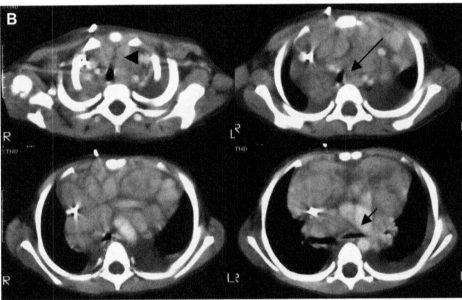

Fig. 7. Lymphoma. A 30-month-old girl presenting with stridor. (*A*) Frontal chest radiograph demonstrates a large mediastinal mass with rightward deviation of the trachea (*arrow*). (*B*) A series of axial intravenous contrast-enhanced CT images of the chest show the anterior and middle mediastinal location of a multilobulated mass with displacement and narrowing of the trachea and the proximal left main stem bronchus (*arrow*). Note also bilateral pleural effusions. (*From* Franco A, Mody NS, Meza MP. Imaging evaluation of pediatric mediastinal masses. Radiol Clin N Am 2005;43:333; with permission.)

symptomatic lesions and is favored for asymptomatic cysts to prevent future complications. The approach is either by VATS or lateral thoracotomy depending on the complexity of the cyst and the experience of the surgeon.[16–18]

POSTERIOR MEDIASTINAL MASSES

Posterior mediastinal masses are most often neurogenic tumors in the paravertebralsulcus. Neurogenic tumors in children have a much higher rate of

malignancy than in adults. These tumors may arise from the sympathetic ganglia (ganglioma, ganglioneuroblastoma, and neuroblastoma), the intercostal nerves (neurofibroma, neurilemoma, and neurosarcoma) and the paraganglia cells (paraganglioma).

Ganglion Tumors

The tumors of the autonomic ganglia—ganglioneuroma, ganglioneuroblastoma and neuroblastoma—represent a continuum of differentiation

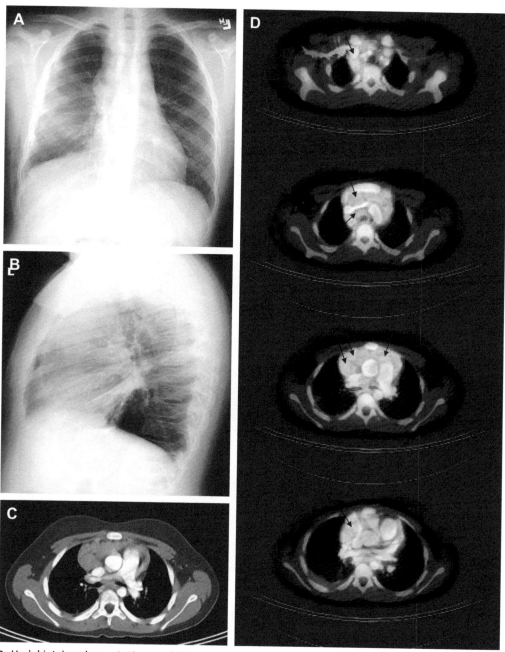

Fig. 8. Hodgkin's lymphoma. A 12-year-old boy presenting with cough. (*A*) Frontal chest radiograph shows a lobular right paratracheal mediastinal silhouette. (*B*) Lateral radiograph demonstrates the anterior location, based on filling in of the clear space with soft tissue. (*C*) Axial contrast-enhanced CT image confirms a right-sided anterior mediastinal lobulated mass. (*D*) A series of PET-CT images show intense activity at numerous levels (*arrows*). (*From* Franco A, Mody NS, Meza MP. Imaging evaluation of pediatric mediastinal masses. Radiol Clin N Am 2005;43:334; with permission.)

and malignancy. Ganglioneuromas are found in the older pediatric population and are the most common pediatric neurogenic tumor. They are composed of ganglion cells and nerve fibers and they are well encapsulated. CT usually demonstrates an encapsulated, relatively homogeneous tumor, occasionally with areas of cystic degeneration. MR is very helpful to define the relationship with the spine, neural foramen, and the spinal cord. They are benign tumors cured with

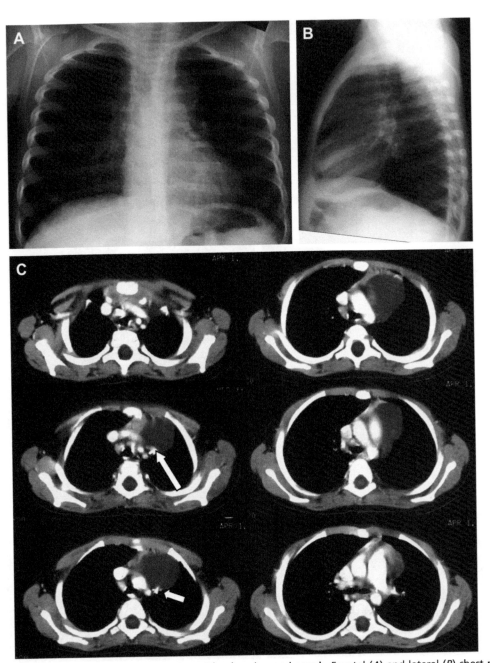

Fig. 9. Teratoma. A 2-year-old boy presenting with wheezing and cough. Frontal (*A*) and lateral (*B*) chest radiographs demonstrate the left anterior mediastinal location of a mass. (*C*) A series of intravenous contrast-enhanced axial CT images illustrated the prominently cystic nature of the mass. Internal calcification is also noted (*arrows*). (*From* Franco A, Mody NS, Meza MP. Imaging evaluation of pediatric mediastinal masses. Radiol Clin N Am 2005;43:335; with permission.)

resection, which can be either by lateral thoracotomy or by VATS.[19,20] They are usually asymptomatic.

Ganglioneuroblastomas represent an intermediate tumor that is malignant. They occur in older children than neuroblastomas and present in a less aggressive fashion. About one half present with symptoms. They are composed of mature and immature ganglion cells and are divided into two varieties: composite and diffuse ganglioneuroblastoma. Composite ganglioneuroblastomas are composed of mature neuroblasts with focal areas

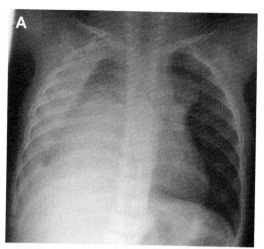

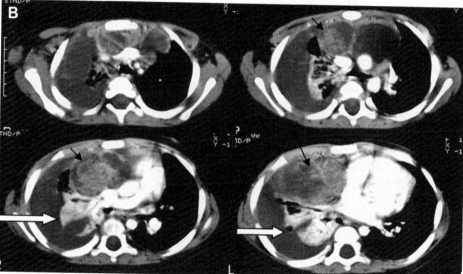

Fig.10. Endodermal sinus tumor.An 18-month-old boy presenting with progressive respiratory distress. (*A*) Frontal chest radiograph shows an abnormal contour at the right heart margin, a mass in the region of the aorticopulmonary window, and a large right effusion. (*B*) A series of axial intravenous contrast-enhanced CT images shows cystic and soft-tissue components (*black arrows*) in addition to the large malignant right pleural effusion and enhancing, atelectatic right lung (*white arrows*). (*From* Franco A, Mody NS, Meza MP. Imaging evaluation of pediatric mediastinal masses. Radiol Clin N Am 2005;43:336; with permission.)

of more primitive neuroblasts. Resection is performed for encapsulated tumors, whereas multimodality therapy similar to neuroblastoma is used for advanced stages. Reports have indicated a prognosis better than and similar to neuroblastoma. Stage is likely the most important determinant of survival. The absence of amplification of MYCN was related to a better prognosis. Five-year survival rates of 88% and 84% have been reported.[21–23]

Neuroblastoma is the most common non–CNS malignant tumor in children. About two thirds of cases are retroperitoneal and one third are mediastinal. They are highly malignant. Most are found in children under the age of three. Metastatic

disease is usually present at the time of diagnosis. Most patients are symptomatic with presentations including dyspnea, chest pain, paraplegia, Horner's syndrome, fever, and weakness. Many different paraneoplastic syndromes can be produced by these tumors. An unusual syndrome, known as opsoclonus–myoclonus syndrome, characterized by rapid involuntary eye movements can be caused by neuroblastomas. Common metastatic sites include the regional nodes, bone, brain, liver, and lung. Neuroblastomas are composed of small round immature ganglion cells often organized in a rosette pattern. Areas of necrosis and calcification are often present. CT examination demonstrates a soft tissue invasive tumor in the

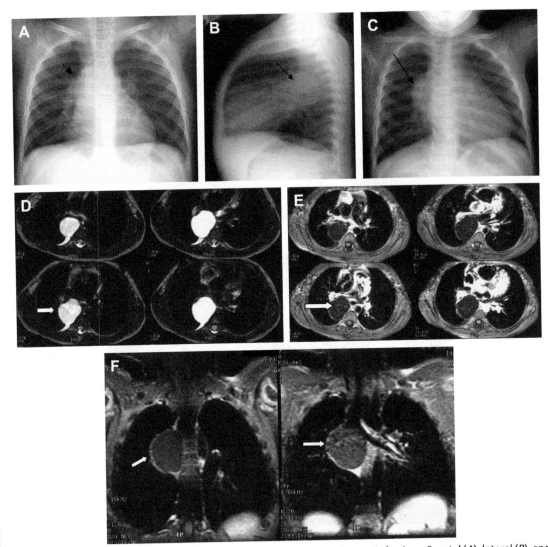

Fig. 11. Bronchogenic cyst. A 2-year-old girl with a history of upper respiratory infections. Frontal (*A*), lateral (*B*), and oblique (*C*) chest radiographs show a rounded middle mediastinal mass (*arrows*). MR images consisting of axial T2-weighted (*D*) and axial (*E*) and coronal (*F*) postcontrast T1-weighted sequences with fat saturation demonstrate the cystic nature of this mass (*arrows*) predominantly in the middle mediastinum. (*From* Franco A, Mody NS, Meza MP. Imaging evaluation of pediatric mediastinal masses. Radiol Clin N Am 2005;43:340; with permission.)

paraspinal mediastinal compartment. There are often areas of necrosis, hemorrhage, and calcification (**Figs. 13** and **14**). MR is very helpful in delineating the extent of chest wall and spinal involvement. About one third of neuroblastomas extend into the neural foramen and spinal canal. Neuroblastomas are staged from I to IV: Stage 1) well-circumscribed tumor with negative nodes; Stage IIA) unilateral tumor, incomplete resection with negative nodes; Stage IIB) unilateral tumor with ipsilateral regional nodal involvement; Stage III) extension of tumor across the midline with or without nodal involvement; Stage IVS) localized primary tumor, children < 1 year of age with metastases limited to liver, skin or bone marrow (not cortical bone, < 10%); Stage IV) widespread distant metastatic disease. Stage I and II tumors are treated by resection; stage III tumors are treated with multimodality therapy and resection; and stage IV tumors are treated with multimodality therapy, sometimes with resection. The role of resection in stage IVS neuroblastomas remains controversial. Age, stage, MYCN status, Shimada histology, and tumor cell ploidy are important prognostic factors. The survival rate of stage I and II tumors is excellent (Stage I, 99%; II, 98%). The survival of stage IVS patients is more variable but still relatively favorable (50%–70%). An

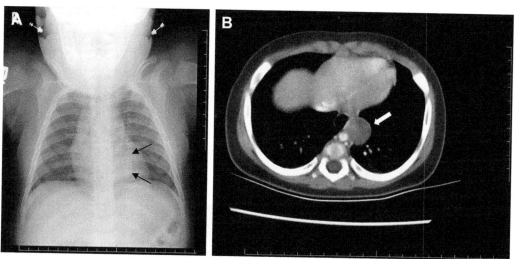

Fig. 12. Esophageal duplication cyst. A 6-year-old girl with a history of chest pain and cough. (*A*) Frontal chest radiograph demonstrates a rounded well-circumscribed opacity (*arrows*). (*B*) Axial intravenous contrast-enhanced CT image at the level of the dome of the liver shows the duplication cyst (*arrow*) located lateral to the esophagus. (*From* Franco A, Mody NS, Meza MP. Imaging evaluation of pediatric mediastinal masses. Radiol Clin N Am 2005;43:341; with permission.)

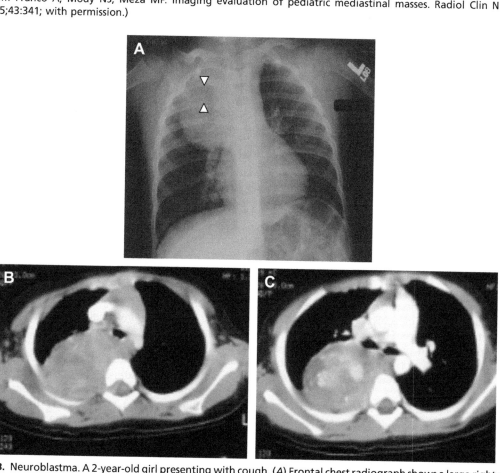

Fig. 13. Neuroblastma. A 2-year-old girl presenting with cough. (*A*) Frontal chest radiograph shows a large right upper mediastinal soft tissue mass. Note the widening of the third to fourth posterior intercostal space (*arrowheads*). (*B*) Intravenous contrast-enhanced axial CT image at the level of the left pulmonary artery shows a mixed attenuation posterior mediastinal mass with extension into the extradural spinal canal. Note that the mass extends across the midline posterior to the trachea. (*C*) Note calcification within the mass. (*From* Franco A, Mody NS, Meza MP. Imaging evaluation of pediatric mediastinal masses. Radiol Clin N Am 2005;43:343; with permission.)

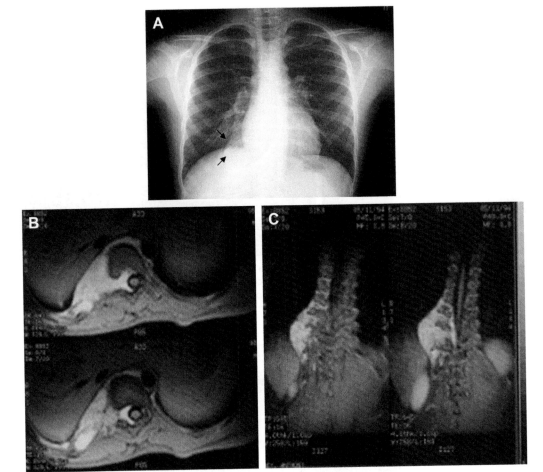

Fig. 14. Neuroblastma. A 9-year-old boy with a history of trauma 11 months previously. The patient presents now with cough and mild chest pain. Multiple prior chest radiographs (not shown) were interpreted as a rightinfrahilar pneumonia. (*A*) Frontal chest radiograph reveals a right medial basilar rounded opacity (*arrows*). (*B, C*) T1-weighted intravenous contrast-enhanced MR images show the abnormality is a brightly enhancing right paraspinal posterior mediastinal mass that extends through the neural formina in to the extradural spinal canal. (*From* Franco A, Mody NS, Meza MP. Imaging evaluation of pediatric mediastinal masses. Radiol Clin N Am 2005;43:346; with permission.)

important study of 141 patients who had stage IV neuroblastoma strongly suggested the importance of resection on freedom from local failure and survival. The incidence of local progression in patients without resection was 50% whereas it was only 10% in those with gross total resection. Overall survival was 50% in patients who had resection and was only 11% in patients who had no resection.[23–25]

Neurofibromas and neurilemonas (Schwannomas) are benign tumors of intercostal or sympathetic nerves. Schwannomas are encapsulated without nerve fibers within the tissue. Neurofibromas are unencapsulated with nerve fibers running through the tissue. Neurofibromas are common in patients with neurofibromatosis. Both are usually asymptomatic and are much more commonly diagnosed in adults as opposed to children. Both are well demarcated on CT, spherical paraspinal masses that are homogeneous. Bone erosion or splaying of the ribs is common. About 10% have intraspinal extension. Resection is curative.

Paraganglioma

Paragangliomas (extra-adrenal pheochromcytoma) are rare tumors of the chromaffin cells of the sympathetic nervous system. Less than 2% of pheochromcytomas occur in the chest. Less than 10% are malignant. Most are encapsulated tumors in the paraspinal location. Patients may present with the signs and symptoms of catecholamine excess. Resection is the treatment of choice. Patients with catecholamine excess need to be medically prepared with alpha and beta adrenergic blockade before operation.[26]

Anesthetic Concerns in Pediatric Mediastinal Tumors

Large anterior mediastinal masses in children may present with airway compromise and yet require anesthesia for either a biopsy or a definitive resection. Loss of the airway or circulatory collapse with induction of general anesthesia has been a well-described scenario in pediatric patients with these large tumors.[27–29] Modern axial CT scans allow an accurate estimation of the degree of airway impingement and facilitate anesthetic and operative planning. Spirometry is useful in older children to assess the functional result of airway compression. Anesthetic techniques used include: inhalational agents with spontaneous ventilation with a laryngeal mask airway; rigid bronchoscopy to provide an airway beyond the compression area; and typical general anesthesia with endotracheal intubation. Most important is preoperative collaboration between the surgeon and anesthesiologist to arrive at a safe perioperative plan for the child.

REFERENCES

1. Takeda S, Miyoshi S, Akinori A, et al. Clinical spectrum of primary mediastinal tumors: A comparison of adult and pediatric populations at a single Japanese institution. J Surg Oncol 2003;83:24–30.
2. Franco A, Mody NS, Meza MP. Imaging evaluation of pediatric mediastinal masses. Radiol Clin North Am 2005;43:325–53.
3. Malone PS, Fitzgerald RJ. Aberrant thymus: a misleading mediastinal mass. J Pediatr Surg 1987;22:130–1.
4. Rice HE, Flake AW, Hori T, et al. Massive thymic hyperplasia: characterization of a rare mediastinal mass. J Pediatr Surg 1994;29:1561–4.
5. Wright CD, Wain JC, Wong DR, et al. Predictors of recurrence in thymic tumors: Importance of invasion, WHO histology and size. J Thorac Cardiovasc Surg 2005;130:1413–21.
6. Cigliano B, Baltogiannis N, De Marco M, et al. Cervical thymic cysts. Pediatr Surg Int 2007;23:1219–25.
7. Glick RD, La Quaglia MP. Lymphomas of the anterior mediastinum. Semin Pediatr Surg 1999;8:69–77.
8. Martino F, Avila LF, Encinas JL, et al. Teratomas of the neck and mediastinum in children. Pediatr Surg Int 2006;22:627–34.
9. Chen CK, Chang YL, Jou ST, et al. Treatment of mediastinal immature teratoma in a child with precocious puberty and Klnefelter'ssysndrome. Ann Thorac Surg 2006;82:1906–8.
10. Billmore DF. Malignant germ cell tumors in childhood. Semin Pediatr Surg 2006;15:30–6.
11. De Backer A, Madern GC, Havkvoort-Cammel FG, et al. Mediastinal germ cell tumors: clinical aspects and outcomes in 7 children. Eur J Pediatr Surg 2006;16:318–22.
12. Okazaki T, Iwatani S, Yani T, et al. Treatment of lymphangioma in children; our experience of 128 cases. J Pediatr Surg 2007;42:386–9.
13. Kavunkal AM, Ramkumar J, Gangahanumiah S, et al. Isolated mediastinal cystic lymphangioma in a child. J Thorac Cardiovasc Surg 2007;134:1596–7.
14. Tan C, Alphonso N, Anderson D, et al. Mediastinal-hemangiomas in children. Eur J Cardiothorac Surg 2003;23:1065–7.
15. Sakurai K, Hara M, Ozawa Y, et al. Thoracic hemangiomas: imaging via CT, MR, and PET along with pathologic correlation. J Thorac imaging 2008;23:114–20.
16. Takda S, Miyoshi S, Minami M, et al. Clinical spectrum of mediastinal cysts. Chest 2003;124:125–32.
17. Michel JL, Revlllon Y, Montupet P, et al. Thoracoscopic treatment of mediastinal cysts in children. J Pediatr Surg 1998;33:1745–8.
18. Meehan JJ, Sandler AD. Robotic resection of mediastinal masses in children. J Laparoendosc Adv Surg Tech A 2008;18:114–9.
19. Nio M, Nakamura M, Yoshida S, et al. Thoracoscopic removal of neurogenicmediastinal tumors in children. J Laparoendosc Adv Surg Tech A 2005;15:80–3.
20. Petty JK, Bensard DD, Patrick DA, et al. Resection of neurogenic tumors in children: is thoracoscopy superior to thoracotomy? J Am Coll Surg 2006;203:699–703.
21. Kubota M, Suita S, Tajiri T, et al. Analysis of prognostic factors relating to better clinical outcome in ganglioneuroblastoma. J Pediatr Surg 2000;35:92–5.
22. Adam A, Hochhlozer L. Ganglioneuroblastoma of the posterior mrdiastinum: a clinicopathologic review of 80 cases. Cancer 1981;47:373–81.
23. Kang CH, Kim YT, Jeon SH, et al. Surgical treatment of malignant mediastinalneurogenic tumors in children. Eur J Cardiothorac Surg 2007;31:725–30.
24. Gutierrez JC, Fischer AC, Sola JE, et al. Markedly improving survival of neuroblastoma: a 30 year analysis of 1,646 patients. Pediatr Surg Int 2007;23:637–46.
25. LaQuaglia MP, Kushner BH, Su W, et al. The impact of gross total resection on local control and survival in high-risk neuroblastoma. J Pediatr Surg 2004;39:412–7.
26. Spector J, Willis D, Ginsburg H. Paraganglioma of the posterior mediastinum: a case report and review of the literature. J Pediatr Surg 2003;38:1114–6.
27. Piastra M, Rugiero A, Caresta E. Life-threatening presentation of mediastinalneoplasm's: report on 7 consecutive pediatric patients. Am J Emerg Med 2005;23:76–82.
28. Hammer GB. Anesthetic management for the child with a mediastinal mass. Paediatr Anaesth 2004;14:95–7.
29. Ricketts RR. Clinical management of anterior mediastinal tumors in children. Semin Pediatr Surg 2001;10:161–8.

Multimodality Treatment of Germ Cell Tumors of the Mediastinum

Kenneth A. Kesler MD[a],*, Lawrence H. Einhorn, MD[b]

KEYWORDS

- Germ cell tumors • Mediastinal tumors
- Nonseminomatous germ cell cancer
- Thoracic surgery • Chemotherapy

Although the majority of germ cell tumors originate in the gonads, 5% to 10% arise within the anterior mediastinum, which represents the second most common site of origin. Various theories have been proposed to explain the pathogenesis of extragonadal germ cell tumors. The most widely accepted theory involves primordial germ cells, which are "misplaced" during embryonic migration through midline structures. Teratoma, one of the "Four Ts" used as a mnemonic for the main differential diagnoses of primary tumors arising in the anterior-mediastinal compartment, actually represents three histologic categories (mature teratoma, seminomatous, and nonseminomatous germ cell tumors) that have distinct biologic behavior. Mature teratomas are the most common germ cell tumor arising in the mediastinum, representing 60% to 70% of all mediastinal germ cell tumors. Mature teratomas are benign, with surgery representing curative therapy. Primary mediastinal seminomas constitute less than half of all malignant primary mediastinal germ cell tumors and have high cure rates with cisplatin-based chemotherapy alone. Nonseminomatous germ cell cancers comprise the main category of the malignant germ cell tumors arising in the mediastinum (PMNSGCT). The treatment of testicular nonseminomatous germ cell tumors with cisplatin-based chemotherapy regimens, followed by surgical resection of residual disease, is considered one of the most successful paradigms of multimodality cancer therapy, with greater than 80% long-term survival.

It has been well established that although histologically similar to their more commonly occurring testicular counterparts, PMNSGCT have a distinctly worse prognosis and therefore have been categorized as "poor risk," along with other subsets of testicular nonseminomatous germ cell tumors.[1] The relatively poorer prognosis is attributed to a different biologic behavior, including the known association with Klinefelter syndrome and the propensity for hematologic dyscrasias, which are not observed in patients with nonseminomatous testicular cancer.[2,3] This article discusses the multimodality treatment strategy for PMNSGCT.

DIAGNOSIS

The vast majority of PMNSGCTs occur in males 20 to 40 years of age, with extremely rare cases of PMNSGCT occurring in females. Most patients present symptomatic with chest pain, cough, superior vena cava syndrome, and shortness of breath secondary to a rapidly growing anterior mediastinal mass. CT scans usually demonstrate a large heterogeneous mass, with occasional evidence of necrosis and hemorrhage.[4] Local invasion into either lung, left bracheocephalic vein, superior vena cava, and pericardium is common, and even direct cardiac chamber or proximal great artery involvement

[a] Department of Surgery, Cardiothoracic Division Indiana University School of Medicine, Indianapolis, IN 46202, USA
[b] Department of Medicine, Hematology/Oncology Division, Indiana University School of Medicine, Indianapolis, IN 46202, USA
* Corresponding author.
E-mail address: kkesler@iupui.edu (K.A. Kesler).

Thorac Surg Clin 19 (2009) 63–69
doi:10.1016/j.thorsurg.2008.09.002
1547-4127/08/$ – see front matter © 2009 Elsevier Inc. All rights reserved.

can occasionally be present. Associated pericardial and pleural effusions are also common but typically not malignant in nature. For any young adult male presenting with a mass in the anterior mediastinal compartment, obtaining serum tumor markers (STM), alpha fetoprotein (AFP) and human chorionic gonadotropin (hCG), is an essential component of clinical evaluation, as significant elevation of either STM is diagnostic for PMNSGCT. Biopsy in these cases is not only unnecessary, but can be misleading because of sampling error within these typically large and heterogeneous neoplasms. Cytologic confirmation with CT-guided fine-needle aspiration is necessary in rare PMNSGCT patients presenting with normal STMs or patients with minor elevations of hCG, which can be present in pure-seminomatous germ cell cancer.

Histologically, these neoplasms are comprised of at least one nonseminmatous germ cell cancer subtype (yolk sac cancer, embryonal carcinoma, or choriocarcinoma in order of frequency), and frequently mixed with some form of teratomatous pathology, ranging from mature teratoma to teratoma with immature elements (stromal atypia), and finally, frank malignant degeneration of teratoma into the so-called "non-germ cell" cancer (sarcomas and epithelial carcinomas).[5]

Metastatic disease is present in 20% to 25% of cases before chemotherapy, with lung being the most common site, followed by neck, liver, bone, and central nervous system (CNS). Chest and abdominal CT scans are standard imaging tests for staging, with other radiologic studies including positron emission tomography (PET) scan and CNS MRI obtained on an individual basis. Gated MRI and echocardiogram can be helpful to determine the presence of great vessel or cardiac involvement, but subtle invasion may not be apparent until postchemotherapy surgical resection is undertaken. A scrotal examination is recommended during evaluation. However, an isolated metastasis to the anterior mediastinum from a testes cancer is distinctly rare in the authors' institution's experience.

CHEMOTHERAPY

After diagnosis and staging, primary surgical therapy for PMNSGCT is inappropriate. PMNSGCTs are usually large and infiltrative neoplasms. Surgical resection as initial therapy will therefore rarely achieve local control and does not treat metastatic disease when present. Appropriate therapy typically begins with cisplatin-based chemotherapy. The combination of BEP (bleomycin, etoposide, and cisplatin) has historically been the standard chemotherapy for poor-risk nonseminomatous

germ cell tumors including PMNSGCT. The relatively lower incidence of benign histology following cisplatin-based chemotherapy for PMSNGCT, as compared with most testicular nonseminomatous germ cell tumors, has prompted exploration of different chemotherapeutic strategies. However, Walsh and colleagues[6] from MD Anderson Hospital reported on 20 PMNSGCT patients who received a very intensive chemotherapy regimen, with eight different agents in various combinations. Although there was high chemotherapy-related morbidity in this series, the 2-year survival rate of 58% was encouraging, particularly because several patients who had failed first-line therapy were included in this study. Subset analysis of 28 PMNSGCT patients from a multicenter phase II German study using high-dose VIP (etoposide, ifosfamide, and cisplatin) with autologous stem-cell rescue for first-line therapy in poor-risk nonseminomatous germ cell tumor patients showed an impressive 68% 2-year overall survival.[7] A recent multi-institutional trial randomized 219 poor-risk nonseminomatous germ cell tumors patients, which included 58 PMNSGCT patients, to either four cycles of standard BEP or two cycles of BEP followed by high-dose carboplatin-based chemotherapy with autologous stem-cell rescue for first-line therapy.[8] Unfortunately, no overall survival advantage was found in the experimental arm in any subset, including the patients with PMNSGCT.

A recent randomized trial comparing BEP to VIP for poor-risk nonseminomatous germ cell tumors including PMNSGCT demonstrated statistically equivalent survival.[9] To eliminate the possibility of bleomycin-induced pulmonary toxicity before a major thoracic surgical procedure, the authors have used VIP combination chemotherapy for the past 2 years. Since initiating this change, the authors' institution has gone from a 14% rate of postoperative pulmonary failure, which carried 50% mortality in these otherwise young and healthy patients after BEP, to no patients experiencing postoperative respiratory failure out of 21 patients to date who received preoperative VIP.

Following chemotherapy, there is typically resolution of pleural and pericardial effusions and a significant decrease in STMs. There is also typically a reduction in tumor dimensions. However, a residual mediastinal mass (RM) is still invariably present. In the authors' and other institutions' experience, the RM pathologically contains complete tumor necrosis only in a distinct minority of cases.[10,11] Therefore, teratoma, persistent nonseminomatous germ cell cancer, and non-germ cell cancer is pathologically present in most RMs for which surgery is indicated. Unfortunately, there is no role for postchemotherapy PET scanning to determine the need for removal of a RM, as teratoma does not demonstrate hypermetabolic activity similar to complete necrosis. PET additionally lacks sensitivity to identify microscopic foci of persistent nonseminomatous germ cell cancer or non-germ cell cancer. Optimally, STMs normalize and surgery is planned after adequate functional and hematologic recovery, which usually occurs between 4 and 6 weeks following completion of chemotherapy.

A controversial area has been the role of surgery in the presence of elevated serum tumor markers following chemotherapy. At the authors' institution a decade ago, PMNSGCT patients with persistently elevated STMs were treated with second-line cisplatin-based chemotherapy before considering surgery, similar to the current treatment paradigm for testicular nonseminomatous germ cell tumors. While second-line cisplatin-based chemotherapy has a 50% "salvage" rate for nonseminomatous germ cell tumors arising in the testes, there has been a very poor response rate for PMNSGCTs.[12] Additionally, there unfortunately appears to be relatively poor sensitivity and specificity of STMs after chemotherapy to detect pathologic evidence of residual viable malignancy in PMNSGCT patients. In a recent study from the authors' institution involving 166 PMNSGCT patients who underwent postchemotherapy resection of residual disease, elevation of either STM was present in 39% patients at the time of surgery.[13] However, only 57% of these patients pathologically demonstrated evidence of malignancy, with either persistent nonseminomatous germ cell cancer or pure non-germ cell cancer. Even 39 patients who presented to surgery with rising STMs had just a 67% chance of pathologically demonstrating persistent nonseminomatous germ cell cancer in the RM. In this study, all but only eight patients with either AFP or hCG levels greater than 1,000 uniformly demonstrated pathologic evidence of persistent nonseminomatous germ cell cancer. Forty-three percent of patients with elevated STMs at the time of surgery, therefore, pathologically demonstrated only benign disease (necrosis/teratoma) and would likely not have benefited from additional chemotherapy. In contrast, 32% of patients with normal STMs at the time of surgery demonstrated pathologic evidence of viable malignancy in the RM, with either persistent nonseminomatous germ cell cancer or pure non-germ cell cancer. Given the historically poor response of second-line chemotherapy, the imperfect correlation of postchemotherapy STM levels to pathologic findings, and the ability for surgery to "salvage" patients with residual malignancy, the authors have subscribed to the policy of surgically removing any residual disease if deemed resectable after first-line cisplatin-based chemotherapy, regardless of STM status.[10,14,15] The authors do believe that two additional cycles of adjuvant cisplatin-based chemotherapy should be considered after recovery if there is pathologic evidence of viable nonseminomatous germ cell cancer in the surgical specimen and the patient had demonstrated response to first-line cisplatin-based therapy.

Occasionally, PMNSGCT patients will demonstrate the so-called "growing teratoma syndrome," with paradoxical growth of a mediastinal mass associated with a rapid decrease of STMs during chemotherapy.[16] The authors agree that chemotherapy should be discontinued and surgery undertaken if feasible in these situations. Of note however, although teratoma is pathologically identified in many of these cases, 57% of patients presenting for surgery at the authors' institution with this clinical scenario have pathologically demonstrated areas of nongerm-cell cancer or even occasionally persistent nonseminomatous germ-cell cancer in the RM.[10] Approximately 5% of patients with PMNSGCT will, unfortunately, demonstrate progressive serologic and radiographic disease during or shortly after first-line chemotherapy and are considered poorly operable to inoperable. The authors are currently investigating the use of high-dose carboplatin-based chemotherapy with tandem stem cell transplant in these cases.

SURGERY

The basic premise of the authors' surgical approach involves a complete en-bloc removal of the RM, thymus, and surrounding involved structures. An approach (sternotomy, posteriorlateral thoracotomy, bilateral anterior thoracotomies with transverse sternotomy or the "clam shell" incision) is planned based on size and location of the RM.[17,18] Cardiopulmonary bypass circuits are routinely available in case cardiac or great vessel involvement is encountered, requiring bypass support. Surgery for PMNSGCT is technically demanding, as preoperative chemotherapy renders surrounding mediastinal tissues fibrotic, obscuring normal anatomic planes. The effectiveness of cisplatin-based chemotherapy for germ cell cancer, however, also usually results in extensive tumor necrosis that is more marked around the periphery. This finding usually allows a complete resection, which minimizes operative morbidity by preserving critical structures that abut but are not densely adherent to or directly involved with the RM, such as lung, great veins, phrenic nerves, and occasionally cardiac chambers where the pericardial barrier has been violated. An extrapleural dissection is considered sufficient if the RM abuts but does not invade the chest wall. If the RM is simply adherent to the visceral pleura of either lung without invasion, removing a small rim of lung parenchyma with the RM is usually adequate to obtain a tumor-free margin. Frank invasion of the RM into pulmonary parenchyma or hilum usually requires formal anatomic resection. Similarly, phrenic nerves can usually be separated from an adjacent RM with scalpel dissection, although dense adherence or direct involvement requires en bloc removal. Diaphragmatic plication is performed only if an ipsilateral lobectomy or pneumonectomy is not required with phrenic nerve resection. If only one (usually the left) bracheocephalic vein is removed en-bloc with the RM, venous reconstruction is usually not performed, as upper extremity venous insufficiency in these cases is typically temporary and minor. If both bracheocephalic veins are removed with the RM, then unilateral bracheocephalic reconstruction, preferably the right, is performed using an externally-stented polytetrafluoroethylene vascular prosthesis. The superior vena cava is similarly reconstructed with externally-stented polytetrafluoroethylene vascular prosthesis, and autologous pericardium is used to patch partial superior vena cava defects. Right atrial and partial pulmonary artery defects are repaired with thin-walled polytetrafluoroethylene prosthetic patches. Intraoperative frozen section analyses of surgical margins are obtained in cases where critical structures abutting the RM are preserved or visibly close surgical margins exist. When required, the timing of pulmonary metastastectomy is individualized, based on several factors, including the surgical approach to the RM, the magnitude of pulmonary resection required to remove the RM, and the magnitude of pulmonary resection required for metastastectomy.

In the authors' recently published surgical experience involving 158 PMNSGCT patients, a sternotomy was used to remove residual disease in 50%, "clam-shell" incision in 27%, and posterior lateral thoracotomy in 23% of the cases, respectively.[10] Adjacent organs removed en bloc with the RM in this series are shown in **Table 1**. The pericardium was the most common adjacent organ adherent to or frankly involved with the RM. As there is no appreciable morbidity from pericardial resection, no attempt was made at separating the RM from the pericardium, which was removed en bloc in 117 patients, typically with a 1-cm to 2-cm tumor-free margin. En bloc pulmonary resection was required in 56% patients. Lobectomy and pneumonectomy were performed in 50 and 9 cases, respectively, with the remainder of patients

Table 1
Organs removed en bloc

Pericardium	117 (74.1)
Lung	88 (55.7)
Wedge/segment	29 (18.4)
Lobectomy	50 (31.6)
LU	33
RU±M13	
Pneumonectomy	9 (5.7)
Left	6
Right	3
Phrenic nerve	50 (31.6)
Great vein	39 (24.7)
Left BC	31
Right BC/SVC	19
Cardiac chamber	6 (3.8)
Right atrium	4
Diaphragm	4 (2.5)
Separate metastatectomy	
Pulmonary	19 (12.0)
Non pulmonary	16 (10.1)

Adjacent organs removed en bloc with the RM and metastatic resections after cisplatin-based chemotherapy in 158 PMNSGCT patients. Number of patients given with percentage of series in parenthesis.
Abbreviations: BC, bracheocephalic; LU, left upper; RU ± M, right upper with or without middle, SVC, superior vena cava.
From Kesler KA, Rieger KM, Hammoud ZT, et al. A 25-year single institution experience with surgery for primary mediastinal nonseminomatous germ cell tumors. Ann Thorac Surg 2008;85:373; with permission.

undergoing sublobar resections. The ipsilateral phrenic nerve was removed with the RM in 50 patients. A great vein was excised with the RM in 39 patients and prosthetic venous reconstruction performed in 10 of these cases. Two patients underwent patch repair of a superior vena cava defect. Cardiopulmonary bypass was required in six patients; four of these required excision and patch repair of the right atrial free wall and two underwent patch repair of the main pulmonary artery. Nineteen patients required pulmonary metastatectomy and 16 patients have undergone staged extrathoracic metastatectomy for either synchronous or metachronous disease including bone ($n = 5$), cervical lymph node ($n = 4$), and central nervous system ($n = 3$).

To decrease the risk of pulmonary complications, efforts are made to minimize intravenous fluid administration and oxygen levels during and immediately after surgery, particularly for patients who have received bleomycin. The vast majority of postchemotherapy nonseminomatous germ cell tumor patients will present to surgery with a baseline sinus tachycardia, which is not treated with fluid or pharmacologic blockade if blood pressure and urine output remain adequate. Patients who presented to surgery with elevated STMs have STMs measured before hospital discharge and at a 1-month follow-up visit. The authors' routine long-term follow-up includes chest radiographs and STMs on an every 6-month basis for the first 5 years, then yearly thereafter for most patients. For patients pathologically demonstrating a component of teratoma, the authors additionally use CT imaging during follow-up, as surgery for early recurrence of teratoma has a high success rate. In contrast, teratoma, particularly with immature elements, has a propensity to degenerate into malignant histology over time, which carries a significantly worse prognosis despite aggressive surgery.

SURVIVAL

It is well established that the overall survival outcome after multimodality treatment of PMNSGCTs is inferior when compared with nonseminomatous germ cell tumors originating in the testes. Goss and colleagues[19] reported on a 14-year experience in Toronto with 24 PMNSGCT patients, and found a 47% survival at 5 years. A multicenter retrospective study from Spain, involving 27 PMNSGCT patients, reported a 32% 5-year survival; however, 12 of these patients had metastatic disease at the time of presentation.[20] Fizazi and colleagues[21] reviewed 38 PMNSGCT patients, 29 of whom were referred for primary treatment to their institution. Only 10 of these patients have remained disease-free after a median follow-up of 89 months. Inferior survival has been mainly attributed to a higher incidence of cisplatin-refractory nonseminomatous germ cell cancer, including

degenerative non-germ cell cancer present in PMNSGCT, as compared with testes nonseminomatous germ cell tumors. Other factors include the propensity of PMNSGCT patients to develop hematologic malignancies, which are usually fatal.[3,22]

The authors have found that the worst pathology identified in the RM following chemotherapy is independently predictive of long-term survival (**Fig. 1**).[10,14] Patients who pathologically demonstrate complete tumor necrosis with no evidence of teratoma or viable cancer have an excellent long-term prognosis, with only a rare late death secondary to recurrent disease. In the authors' series, patients with pathologic evidence of teratoma, with or without tumor necrosis, demonstrate intermediate survival. Although considered benign, teratoma in PMNSGCT cases not infrequently contain immature elements. When present, occult teratoma metastases therefore do have potential to degenerate into malignant histology. "Salvage" surgical therapy, where viable nonseminomatous germ cell cancer or non-germ cell cancer are pathologically identified in the RM, results in relatively worse but possible long-term survival, even in the face of rising STMs.[23] From institutional data, patients with less than 50% of the RM containing viable malignancy have an approximate 50% long-term survival following aggressive surgery, which is diminished when greater than or equal to 50% of the RM contains viable malignancy (**Fig. 2**). Other reports have also found heterogeneous survival for PMNSGCT patients. The Memorial Sloan Kettering Cancer Center reported a series of 49 PMNSGCT patients, 32 of whom underwent surgical resection of residual disease after platin-based chemotherapy.[11] Complete tumor necrosis was identified in 12% of surgical specimens, where teratoma and viable cancer were found in 66%. The overall 2-year survival for their series was 38%. However, an 81%

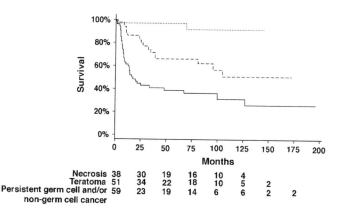

Fig. 1. Long-term survival based on worst pathologic category identified in the RM after cisplatin-based chemotherapy and complete surgery. The pathologic category was independently predictive of survival by multivariable analysis. Numbers represent patients at risk. Necrosis shown by dotted line; teratoma shown by interrupted line; Persistent germ cell cancer or non-germ cell cancer shown by solid line. (*From* Kesler KA, Rieger KM, Hammoud ZT, et al. A 25-year single institution experience with surgery for primary mediastinal nonseminomatous germ cell tumors. Ann Thorac Surg 2008;85:374; with permission.)

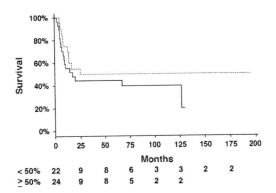

| < 50% | 22 | 9 | 8 | 6 | 3 | 3 | 2 | 2 |
| ≥ 50% | 24 | 9 | 8 | 5 | 2 | 2 | | |

Fig. 2. A trend toward improved long-term when the amount of viable persistent germ-cell cancer or non-germ cell cancer was less than 50% of the RM (*dotted line*) as compared with 50% or greater (*solid line*). Numbers represent patients at risk. (*From* Kesler KA, Rieger KM, Hammoud ZT, et al. A 25-year single institution experience with surgery for primary mediastinal nonseminomatous germ cell tumors. Ann Thorac Surg 2008;85:374; with permission.)

survival rate was found in patients demonstrating pathology of necrosis or teratoma. A large multicenter review of extragonadal nonseminomatous germ-cell tumor patients, including 287 with PMNSGCT, reported an overall 5-year survival of 45%.[24] Two year survival varied widely in this study, from 34% in the subset of patients who presented visceral metastases to 84% in younger patients without metastases and normal hCG at the time of diagnosis. Only 49% of PMNSGCT patients underwent postchemotherapy surgery in this review. Teratoma and complete necrosis was present in 26% and 37% of patients, respectively; however, the pathology of any excised residual disease was not analyzed with respect to survival outcome.

SUMMARY

Germ cell tumors originating in the anterior mediastinal compartment represent a rare but biologically interesting group of neoplasms. Knowledge of the specific biologic behaviors and therapeutic strategies for the three histologic types is important. PMNSGCT represent the most challenging group of malignant germ cell tumors and survival outcome is dependant on both successful chemotherapy and surgery to remove residual disease when feasible. The authors currently believe non-bleomycin-containing regimens will reduce operative risks in this regard. New chemotherapy strategies that reduce the incidence of persistent nonseminatous germ cell or non-germ cell cancer

need continued investigation. Although overall survival is inferior to nonseminomatous germ cell tumors of testicular origin, favorable subsets with pathologic evidence of either necrosis or teratoma have been identified. An aggressive surgical approach after cisplatin-based chemotherapy can result in long-term survival, even in patients with persistent nonseminomatous germ cell or non-germ cell cancer, and is warranted in these otherwise young and healthy patients.

REFERENCES

1. International Germ Cell Consensus Classification: a prognostic factor-based staging system for metastatic germ cell cancers. International Germ Cell Cancer Collaborative Group. J Clin Oncol 1997;15: 594–603.
2. Nichols CR, Heerema NA, Palmer C, et al. Klinefelter's syndrome associated with mediastinal germ cell neoplasms. J Clin Oncol 1987;5:1290–4.
3. Nichols CR, Roth BJ, Heerema NA, et al. Hematologic neoplasia associated with mediastinal germ cell neoplasms. N Engl J Med 1990;322:1425–9.
4. Strollo DC, Rosado de Christenson ML, Jett JR. Primary mediastinal tumors part I: tumors of the anterior mediastinum. Chest 1997;112:511–22.
5. Reuter V. The pre and post chemotherapy pathologic spectrum of germ cell tumors. Chest Surg Clin N Am 2002;12:673–94.
6. Walsh GL, Taylor GD, Nesbitt JC, et al. Intensive chemotherapy and radical resections for primary nonseminomatous mediastinal germ cell tumors. Ann Thorac Surg 2000;69:337–43.
7. Bokemeyer C, Schleucher N, Metzner B, et al. First-line sequential high-dose VIP chemotherapy with autologous transplant for patients with primary mediastinal nonseminomatous germ cell tumours: a prospective trial. Br J Cancer 2003;89:29–35.
8. Motzer RJ, Nichols CJ, Margolin KA, et al. Phase III randomized trial of conventional-dose chemotherapy with or without high-dose chemotherapy and autologous hematopoietic stem-cell rescue as first-line treatment for patients with poor-prognosis metastatic germ cell tumors. J Clin Oncol 2007;25(3): 247–56.
9. Hinton S, Catalano P, Einhorn L, et al. Cisplatin, etoposide and either bleomycin or ifosfamide in the treatment of disseminated germ cell tumors: final analysis of an intergroup trial. Cancer 2003;97: 1869–75.
10. Kesler KA, Rieger KM, Hammoud ZT, et al. A 25-year single institution experience with surgery for primary mediastinal nonseminomatous germ cell tumors. Ann Thorac Surg 2008;85:371–8.
11. Vuky J, Bains M, Bacik J, et al. Role of postchemotherapy adjunctive surgery in the management of

patients with nonseminoma arising from the mediastinum. J Clin Oncol 2001;19:682–8.

12. Hartmann J, Einhorn L, Nichols C, et al. Second-line chemotherapy in patients with relapsed extragonadal non-seminomatous germ cell tumors: results of an international multicenter analysis. J Clin Oncol 2001;19:1641–8.

13. Kruter LE, Kesler KA, Yu M, et al. The predictive value of serum tumor markers for pathologic findings of residual mediastinal masses after chemotherapy for primary mediastinal nonseminomatous germ cell tumors [abstract]. Proceedings of the American Society of Clinical Oncology 2008;5087.

14. Kesler K, Rieger K, Ganjoo K, et al. Primary mediastinal nonseminomatous germ cell tumors: the influence of postchemotherapy pathology on long-term survival after surgery. J Thorac Cardiovasc Surg 1999;18:692–700.

15. Schneider B, Kesler K, Brooks J, et al. Outcome of patients with residual germ cell or non-germ cell malignancy after resection of primary mediastinal nonseminomatous germ cell cancer. J Clin Oncol 2004;2:1195–200.

16. Afifi H, Bosl G, Burt M. Mediastinal growing teratoma syndrome. Ann Thorac Surg 1997;64:359–62.

17. Kesler KA, Germ cell tumors of the mediastinum. Chapter 132. In: Pearson FG, et al, editors. Thoracic Surgery. 3rd edition. Churchill Livingstone, Elsevier; 2008.

18. Wright C, Kesler KA. Surgical techniques and outcomes for primary mediastinal nonseminomatous germ cell tumors. Chest Surg Clin N Am 2002;12:707–15.

19. Goss P, Schwertfeger L, Blackstein M, et al. Extragonadal germ cell tumors: a 14-year Toronto experience. Cancer 1994;73:1971–9.

20. Hidalgo M, Paz-Ares L, Rivera F, et al. Mediastinal nonseminomatous germ cell tumors treated with cisplatin-based combination chemotherapy. Ann Oncol 1997;8:555–9.

21. Fizazi K, Culine S, Droz J, et al. Primary mediastinal nonseminomatous germ cell tumors: Results of modern therapy including cicplatin-based chemotherapy. J Clin Oncol 1998;16:725–32.

22. Hartmann JT, Nichols CR, Droz JP, et al. Hematologic disorders associated with primary mediastinal nonseminomatous germ cell tumors. J Natl Cancer Inst 2000;92:54–61.

23. Radaideh SM, Cook VC, Kesler KA, et al. Outcome following resection for patients with primary mediastinal nonseminomatous germ cell tumors and rising serum tumor markers post-chemotherapy [abstract]. Proceedings of the American Society of Clinical Oncology 2008;5038.

24. Hartmann JT, Nichols CR, Droz J, et al. Prognostic variables for response and outcome in patients with extragondal germ cell tumors. Ann Oncol 2002;13:1017–28.

Multimodality Treatment of Thymic Tumors

Federico Venuta, MD[a,b,*], Erino A. Rendina, MD[c],
Giorgio F. Coloni, MD[d]

KEYWORDS

- Thymoma • Mediastinal tumors
- Superior vena cava syndrome • Chemotherapy
- Radiotherapy • Mulitmodality therapy

Thymic tumors are rare human neoplasms; they account for 50% of the anterior mediastinal masses and are the most frequent in adults.[1,2] These tumors show remarkable clinical and pathologic polymorphisms, with a variable and unpredictable evolution ranging from an indolent noninvasive attitude to a highly infiltrative and metastasizing one. Even patients who have invasive lesions, however, tend to show a prolonged clinical course studded with multiple operations performed for diagnosis, primary resection, and treatment of recurrences alternated to cycles of chemo- radiotherapy. These patients are generally younger and fitter than other groups of patients who have thoracic malignancies (lung, esophagus, pleura). For this reason, treatment can be aggressive; nevertheless, in many cases, long-term survival does not correspond to cure and disease-free survival.

Numerous prognostic variables have been considered to predict and interpret the clinical course of these patients: the association with myasthenia gravis and other immunologic disorders, age, invasion of the great vessels, tumor diameter, and onset of recurrence.[2–6] The role of histology was long debated until the new histogenetic classifications were developed.[7–10] The World Health Organization (WHO) classification[1,11,12] now should be included among the independent prognostic factors. Because surgery long was considered the mainstay of treatment, however, prognosis was established to correspond mainly to completeness of resection and Masaoka staging.[2,13–17] Complete surgical resection certainly allows better survival but does not eliminate the incidence of recurrence. For this reason, radiotherapy and chemotherapy have been added to surgical resection in an attempt to improve outcome for patients who have invasive lesions; however, they have not effectively contributed to achieve cure. For this reason, although large multicenter studies are not yet available, new concepts concerning the clinical approach to invasive thymic tumors are emerging as a result of non-standardized multimodality protocols based on single-center experiences. This approach is intended in two forms often associated one to the other:

> Neoadjuvant (induction) chemotherapy administered before surgery to reduce the bulk of the tumor, local invasiveness, and potentially favoring downstaging; it should allow at least a higher rate of complete resections
>
> Adjuvant chemo-radiotherapy after surgery in both R0 and R+ patients who have invasive tumors to reduce the local and distant recurrence rate during follow up

This combined approach (induction, surgery, adjuvant) should allow long- term disease-free survival and cure.

[a] Department of Thoracic Surgery, University of Rome Sapienza, Policlinico Umberto I, Rome, Italy
[b] Lung Transplantation Unit, University of Rome Sapienza, Policlinico Umberto I, Rome, Italy
[c] Thoracic Surgery Unit, University of Rome Sapienza, Ospedale S. Andrea, Rome, Italy
[d] Thoracic Surgery Unit, Department of Surgery, University of Rome Sapienza, Policlinico Umberto I, Rome, Italy
* Corresponding author.
E-mail address: federico.venuta@uniroma1.it (F. Venuta).

Thorac Surg Clin 19 (2009) 71–81
doi:10.1016/j.thorsurg.2008.09.008
1547-4127/08/$ – see front matter © 2009 Elsevier Inc. All rights reserved.

HOW TO PLAN TREATMENT
Staging, Histology, and Other Prognostic Factors

Every classification or staging system has the clear purpose of predicting the clinical course and prognosis of the disease; this helps to design the most appropriate treatment for each patient. Clinical staging long has been considered and validated as the only variable able to predict outcome for patients who have thymic tumors. Many staging systems have been proposed in the past,[2,15,18] and also an attempt to employ the TNM classification was performed without success.[19–21] The only classification that has gained widespread acceptance and stood the test of time is the one proposed by Masaoka and colleagues[15] in 1981 and subsequently modified in 1994.[21] This classification is divided into five stages:

> **Stage I**—macroscopically and microscopically completely encapsulated
> **Stage IIA**—microscopic transcapsular invasion
> **Stage IIB**—macroscopic invasion into the surrounding mediastinal fat tissue or grossly adherent to but not through the mediastinal pleura
> **Stage III**—invasion into the neighboring organs
> **Stage IVA**—pleural or pericardial dissemination
> **Stage IVB**—lymphogenous or hematogenous metastases

The Masaoka classification is based on the evidence of microscopic and macroscopic invasion into the capsule of the tumor and adjacent mediastinal fat and structures. The assumption that led to this classification was that local aggressiveness (even microscopic invasion of the capsule) could make a difference in the clinical course of these patients. Metastatic spread occurs less often than in other tumors and is directed predominantly to the pericardium and pleura, and occasionally to the lung. Extrathoracic dissemination and lymphogenous spread through the regional lymph nodes are possible, although unusual at the time of presentation. Although this staging system has been validated repeatedly, there remain some controversies that could bear on the design of the most appropriate therapeutic program for each patient.

Thymomas often are capsulated, and just for this reason many of them have been called benign thymoma independently from the clinical course. Some of these capsulated and apparently indolent lesions, however, show cytologic and histologic features identical to those of invasive malignant thymomas (identified as stage 3 and 4 according to the Masaoka classification) and lately develop

recurrence. For these reasons, it is not accurate enough to assess prognosis and plan treatment only on the basis of clinical staging; if only this variable is considered as a prognostic factor, it may misinterpret the true nature of the lesion, especially at early stages, underestimating the potential growth, recurrence, and onset of metastases. In fact, despite the indolent behavior repeatedly stressed when reporting on these lesions, recurrence and metastases have been observed in all large series after resection.[9,21–26] This is true even for stage 1 thymomas[6,16,21–33] and for each histologic subtype,[16,21–23,27,29,33–36] even if some authors demonstrated the lack of recurrence in some histologic types (medullary or type A).[9,10,26,37–40] For this reason, other variables should be considered along with staging, matching all the information when assessing prognosis.

The histologic classifications failed to reach a significant prognostic value for a long time, until the modern histogenetic model was adopted. The problem concerning the value of histology also was related to the fact that morphology was usually available only after surgery; thus, most of the management decisions traditionally have been made by preoperative radiological work up and clinical staging. Histology only could contribute to give a name to the lesion without any impact on treatment planning. When the modern histogenetic classifications were developed, the weight of this variable on decision making started to change, giving also more space to the need of preoperative tissue diagnosis. In fact, the Marino and Muller Hermelink classification (medullary, cortical, and mixed types),[8,9] and more recently the WHO system,[12] rapidly gained acceptance and were validated repeatedly by multivariate analysis.[14,16,26,40–42] The WHO types are as follows (types listed as synonyms):

> **Type A**—spindle cell thymoma; medullary thymoma
> **Type AB**—mixed thymoma
> **Type B1**—lymphocyte-rich thymoma; lymphocytic thymoma; predominantly cortical thymoma
> **Type B2**—cortical thymoma
> **Type B3**—well-differentiated thymic carcinoma; epithelial thymoma; squamoid thymoma
> **Type C**—thymic carcinoma (heterogeneous)

These classification systems consistently correlated with the Masaoka staging, prognosis, and long-term outcome. The WHO classification now is accepted as the official one and is considered as an independent prognostic variable. From type A to type C (thymic carcinoma), there is a clear deterioration of prognosis. A, AB, B1, and B2 show a progressively worse outcome; B3 (the old "well differentiated carcinoma") is more aggressive and shows intermediate survival, while thymic carcinoma has the worst prognosis. This classification has been proven to be so effective that it contributed to incorporating type C tumors from the category "thymoma."[12,21]

Other prognostic factors have been added over the years. As mentioned before, completeness of resection is a consistent independent prognostic factor. In stage 3 and 4 tumors, the recurrence rate appears to be lower after complete resection when compared with microscopically or grossly incomplete resection.[43] Even survival after partial resection is slightly better than after simple biopsy,[15,24,29,30,44] although this benefit remains debated, because only one study attempted to correct for the stage when comparing partial resection with biopsy.[28] This was one of the studies that reported a substantial difference. Ten-year disease-free survival was significantly higher for partially resected stage 3 and 4 thymomas compared with those undergoing biopsy only (80%, 62%, and 0%, respectively). Also, the dimensions of the tumor (diameter) are considered a reliable prognostic factor: the larger the diameter the higher the probability to have a recurrence.[5]

The presence of myasthenia gravis (MG) no longer is considered a negative prognostic factor[30,41] as in older studies;[45] in fact most of the recent reports have suggested either a trend[23,28,46,47] or significantly better survival in this group of patients when compared with those without MG.[24,31,48] This probably is related to the fact that the presence of MG favors earlier diagnosis of thymoma; in fact, in most of the studies, MG patients had predominantly stage 1 and 2 tumors.[16,22,28,29,49]

An attempt to use lymph node status as a prognostic factor has been reported.[50] Even if lymph node involvement clearly acts as a negative prognostic index, however, the rarity of this presentation (less than 2%) indicates that this factor would not be a good candidate for stratifying survival in a staging system. Still, knowing the lymph node status certainly contributes to staging (Masaoka 4B) and assessment of prognosis.

Involvement of the great vessels has been found to be an independent negative prognostic factor by multivariate analysis.[28] Also, recurrence has been stressed as a poor outcome predictor and is more frequent at advanced stages and with less differentiated histology. All these variables should be considered when planning the most appropriate treatment for each patient.

Where Can One Arrive With Surgery?

Surgical intervention is the most effective treatment modality for thymic tumors; the operation usually is performed through median sternotomy, and the whole thymus and surrounding mediastinal fat should be removed. The operative mortality does not exceed 2% in most of the recent series,[41,46,51–53] even if it should be correlated with the extent of the resection of the surrounding structures.

Up to 40% of the thymic tumors are invasive,[4] and complete resection often is hampered either by extended local infiltration or dissemination outside the mediastinum.[43,54–56] The ability to achieve complete resection is clearly the key factor for cure[23,29] and must be regarded as the gold standard for treatment, especially for advanced- stage lesions. For these reasons, incomplete resection and debulking should be considered a failure, because they offer no advantage over simple biopsy.[23,28,29,31] The ability to perform a grossly and microscopically complete resection varies with the stage of the tumor and the willingness of the individual surgeon to perform an extended resection incorporating the surrounding structures.

Surgery alone is clearly an effective way of curing patients with a completely capsulated tumor. This group of lesions includes stage 1 thymomas that show a nearly 90% 5-year survival and 80% 10-year survival,[24,25,29,33,41] although there are occasional local recurrences. Incomplete resections do not occur at this stage, and additional treatment (radiotherapy) has not shown to increase survival.[57]

Surgery plays a major role also for locally invasive disease. Complete resection clearly helps to improve survival even if extracapsular invasion is present.[58–61] Locally invasive thymomas include stage 2 and 3 lesions. These are two different categories that also should be matched with the WHO classification. In this group of patients (particularly stage 2), thymoma often can be resected completely; however, notwithstanding complete resection, the tumor can recur and metastasize. Stage 2 lesions can be removed easily, even when the capsule and adjacent mediastinal tissue are macroscopically involved; however, also at this stage local recurrence and distant metastases are observed notwithstanding the administration of adjuvant radiotherapy.[41] B2, B3, and C tumors show a higher incidence of recurrence. Stage 3 lesions (invasion of the lung, superior vena cava, innominate vein, pericardium, great vessels, chest wall) require more extended procedures with en bloc resection of the primary tumor and involved structures. In this group of patients, only 50% of the lesions on average can be resected completely; however, there is wide variability (0% to 89%)[4] that may be explained by the different philosophy, judgment, and skills of each surgeon. This is certainly one of the keys for success; however, the reported survival for patients who have advanced disease is unsatisfactory even after complete resection (10-year survival ranging between 35% and 53%, often with adjuvant radiotherapy).[42] Furthermore, up to 50% of patients undergoing surgery at this stage, whether with complete resection or not, will show recurrence within 5 years,[62–64] even if adjuvant therapy is administered (mainly radiotherapy).[5,41,42,62,63] Most of the recurrences will be on the pleura or in the lung.[63]

Surgical treatment of thymic tumors at this stage leaves many open questions:

Can one predict preoperatively the possibility to perform complete resection?

Should one always perform invasive staging (thoracoscopy or anterior mediastinotomy) and obtain histology before planning treatment of invasive lesions?

Can the rate of complete resections be improved?

Do lesions at this stage require induction anyway, independent from resectability, like for other tumors?

Should one be guided only by the stage of the lesion, or should one integrate it with histology?

Should one use different drugs for the different histologic subtypes, in particular for thymic carcinoma?

Also, stage 4A lesions have been included in this controversial field; this stage, although spreading, is confined to the chest and usually poses several problems. Surgery alone is not considered the most effective approach any more. In the original report from Masaoka,[15] patients who had stage 4 (A and B) showed 5-year and 10-year survival of 50% and 0% respectively. Since then, a range of survival rates has been reported for tumors at this stage (from 40% to 78% at 5 years) (**Table 1**).[15,24,62,65,66] Also at this stage, the peculiar clinical course of this disease has left room for very aggressive surgical interventions, like pleuropneumonectomy,[65,66] that were able to significantly improve survival when performed within a multidisciplinary protocol.

Those open questions has led to a spreading of combined approaches tailored on the clinical status of each patient, integrating surgery, chemotherapy, and radiotherapy.

BACKGROUND TO INTEGRATE CHEMOTHERAPY AND RADIOTHERAPY WITH SURGERY

The optimal treatment of patients with thymic tumors should allow disease-free long-term survival and cure. As mentioned before, however, it has been proved that surgery alone may fail to achieve this target. Additional therapy should be administered before and/or after surgery; the former would help to increase the number of complete resections in patients who have advanced stage tumors. They both should help those patients undergoing incomplete resection, those who have metastatic (stage 4A) lesions, or those who have tumors that are

Table 1
Stage 4 thymoma: long-term survival

Author	Year	n	5-Year Survival	10-Year Survival
Masaoka	1981	11	50%	0%
Nakahara	1988	15	47%	47%
Maggi	1991	21	59%	40%
Pan	1994	12	41%	2
Regnard	1996	19	—	30%
Yagi	1996	5	67%	33%
Wilkins	1999	5	40%	40%
Kondo	2003	67	40%	67%
Nakagawa	2003	11	47%	47%
Lucchi	2005	16	—	46%
Wright	2006	5	75%	50%
Huang	2007	18	78%	65%

macroscopically less invasive but show histology and dimensions that predict the potential onset of recurrence. In these subsets, surgery should be integrated by chemotherapy (pre- and postoperative) and radiotherapy. The administration of additional treatment is based on the empiric experience in medical oncology with advanced thymoma. Almost every single center, however, has its own protocol, and there is not yet a standardized consensus with this approach.

Chemotherapy Background

The efficacy of chemotherapy previously was validated in inoperable thymic tumors. Although single agents have demonstrated activity in recurrent, metastatic, and locally advanced disease, combination regimens generally have shown higher response rates and certainly contribute to create the basis for the current multimodality regimens.

Early case reports and small series showed that thymomas are relatively sensitive to several antineoplastic drugs, although most series were retrospective and included small groups of patients. They clearly demonstrated, however, that chemotherapy can shrink the tumor and palliate symptoms[67] with a response rate that approaches an average of 70% in phase 2 studies with combination regimens.[68] Cisplatin is the basis of most of the protocols. In a literature review,[69] an overall response rate of 84% was obtained with regimens containing this drug; however, durable (lasting several months up to 10 years) and consistent (up to 58%) responses have been observed also in patients receiving nonplatinum-containing regimens.[54,70–73] To date, the best results in phase 2 studies have been obtained with the PAC (cisplatin, doxorubicin and cyclophosphamide) and ADOC regimens (cisplatin, doxorubicin, vincristine, and cyclophosphamide) developed by an Italian group,[74] with a higher response rate for the latter association (92% versus 50%) and a comparable median duration of response.[74,75] Also, the association of cisplatin and etoposide[76] showed encouraging overall survival at advanced stages. Isofosfamide showed impressive single-agent activity,[77] but the incorporation of this drug into a cisplatin-based combination chemotherapy regimen did not yield better results than older regimens.[42] There were no complete responses, with a response rate of 32%.

Thymic carcinoma is less responsive to cytotoxic chemotherapy, and its inclusion in many series certainly contributes to decrease overall survival. Patient selection is also important, because the response rate in the disseminated disease setting is lower than the one observed in the group of patients who had locally advanced disease. This is a common observation in medical oncology and is certainly one of the theoretic bases encouraging administration of induction chemotherapy to patients who have stage 3 thymic tumors potentially unsuitable to surgery with complete resection.

Radiotherapy Background

The role of radiation therapy has not been tested in prospective randomized studies; however, this treatment always has been considered as effective as adjuvant therapy for invasive lesions, because these tumors are usually radioresponsive.[78] Many retrospective studies have shown improvement in local control and survival with adjuvant radiation after surgery for invasive thymoma.[15,29,60,79–81]

There are various dose and fraction schemes reported in the literature,[82] but generally postoperative total doses of 45 to 55 Gy are recommended,[13,44,58,79,83–86] even if there is no clear dose–response relationship because of the paucity of cases and lack of prospective randomized studies. A higher dose (greater than 60 Gy) has been proposed for patients who have bulky disease,[86,87] because lower doses of radiation therapy have been found to adversely affect prognosis.[88]

Primary radiation therapy alone as the definitive treatment was advocated through the early 1990s in nonsurgical candidates or in patients who had unresectable or advanced disease (stages 3 and 4). Results were viable and not comparable, with a 5-year survival that was even higher than 85% in a small group of patients who had stage 4A disease treated with radiotherapy alone.[89]

Preoperative radiotherapy has been employed rarely,[62,90] probably for the fear of the onset of sternal complications after surgery and respiratory complications during the postoperative course. Currently, the role of preoperative and primary radiation therapy has fallen out of interest.

Overall, the improved response rates to chemotherapy and radiotherapy have encouraged their integration with surgery and the treatment of patients with a combined modality approach.

MULTIMODALITY APPROACH

Based on the assumption that invasive thymoma show a relatively high recurrence rate if treated by resection alone and that these tumors respond favorably to both radiation and chemotherapy, many authors have proposed a combined modality approach with the association of the three treatment modalities. Most of the studies focus only on the induction strategy with chemotherapy;

however, a combined modality approach should consider also postoperative consolidation with radiation and chemotherapy.

The appropriate indication to neoadjuvant chemotherapy remains debated; it should be reserved for histologically proven invasive thymoma or thymic carcinoma. Patients should show a good ECOG performance status, normal renal and hepatic functions, and normal hematology and left ventricular function. The disease should be bidimensionally measurable as evaluated by CT scans of the chest. This strategy should allow a higher rate of complete resections. The administration of postoperative treatment should allow better control of the disease even in case of partial resection. It should be administered to those patients receiving induction, but also to those preoperatively deemed completely resectable, and thus not receiving induction chemotherapy. Adjuvant treatment should be administered both in case of complete and incomplete resection and should include chemo- and radiotherapy when the clinical status of the patient allows it. The combined modality treatment should allow prevention of local and distant recurrence and eventually long-term survival with cure. These regimens have been tolerated well, and the results appear better than historical controls, because prospective studies are extremely rare and randomization is virtually nonexistent. Also a small subset of stage 2 tumors should receive postoperative treatment.

When approaching this strategy, different subsets of patients should be considered:

  Stage 3 tumors preoperatively considered not completely resectable
  Stage 3 tumors completely resected with or without induction therapy
  Stage 3 tumors deemed resectable before surgery but incompletely resected
  Stage 4 tumors
  Stage 2 tumors

The philosophy of the different centers when facing each of these categories is slightly different, even if a more uniform approach is gaining acceptance.

Because the true novelty of the combined approach is induction therapy, some general considerations should be made. Preoperative chemotherapy regimens have been tolerated well, and most patients arrive in good conditions for surgery. This is because patients who have thymoma represent a group completely different from those who have other thoracic malignancies. They are younger, fitter, show fewer comorbidities, and can stand much more aggressive regimens. The decision to administer induction therapy is made

preoperatively. In this setting, a correct histologic diagnosis cannot be disregarded, because in the resected specimen, after chemotherapy, there may be only fibrosis, with no pathologic tissue; this finding has been observed in approximately 20% of the patients[2] with a maximum of 44%.[91] Furthermore, the possibility to diagnose thymoma only on the basis of the radiological appearance, although feasible,[2] may present some difficulties, and lymphoma or germ cell tumors could be misdiagnosed with invasive thymoma.

A second point that should be addressed concerns the administration of induction chemotherapy in patients who have thymus-related syndromes, and in particular MG. Chemotherapy usually is tolerated well by these patients, and no deterioration was observed in the authors' experience[41,42] or by other authors.[51,84,91–93] Some partial remissions were observed;[91] this is additional evidence of the efficacy of chemotherapy on thymic tumors and may represent an adjunctive tool to monitor response[71] to treatment and bring patients in a better status to surgery.

Preoperative radiotherapy rarely has been used in patients who have stage 3 thymoma.[59,62,90,94,95] The ability to carry out a complete resection in this subset of patients does not differ from the average resectability rate of patients not receiving induction,[2] and survival does not show any benefit. Concerning radiotherapy, however, the modern three-dimensional conformal planning and intensity-modulated radiation therapy allows higher dosages with less toxicity. This technical improvement should be taken into account when evaluating the actual potential of radiotherapy compared with historical controls.

Stage 3 tumors are the group of thymic lesions approached more often with a combined modality treatment. Induction chemotherapy has proven to be effective in patients who have potentially unresectable lesions; it allows a higher incidence of complete resections and reduces the recurrence rate, improving survival.[41,42,51,91–93] All the induction regimens are cisplatinum-based; the associated drugs vary from study to study, including more frequently cyclophosphamide, doxorubicin, vincristine, etoposide, or epirubicin. Three cycles usually are administered preoperatively.

This approach has not been validated as an independent prognostic factor, even if some benefit in terms of long-term survival has been reported.[42,51,91–93] The authors' policy is to deliver induction therapy only to patients who have bulky aggressive tumors deemed unresectable or not completely resectable at preoperative work-up. Preoperative judgment of resectability of invasive mediastinal lesions greatly depends of the experience and technical skills of each surgeon; tumors considered resectable by someone could be judged unresectable by others. For this reason, invasive staging, with all the limitations of this approach, should be considered to facilitate decision making.[41] Preinduction invasive staging should be recommended, and in the authors' experience, it never has favored seeding within the pleural space or through the thoracoscopic port.[41,42] Limited invasion of the superior vena cava or the lung should not be considered an indication for induction therapy. The indications for this approach should be reserved to tumors with a more extended involvement of the mediastinum and no evident cleavage plans, to bulky lesions abutting and invading both mediastinal sides, with extended invasion of the vessels, the lung, and the chest wall. In this subset of patients, many groups[41,51,84,91,92,96] reported a reliable complete response rate (up to 44%); downstaging also was observed in some cases.[41,92,96]

In this group of patients, treatment should be completed with postoperative consolidation chemotherapy (two to three additional cycles) and 50 to 60 Gy of radiotherapy over the site of the primary lesion (both in case of complete and incomplete resection).[41,42,84,91,92,96] Consolidation therapy is mandatory in case of positive lymph nodes; for this reason, lymph nodes at least should be sampled during the operation. It has been reported that completeness of resection loses statistical significance in the cohort of patients receiving the combined approach (pre- and postoperative).[92] This finding has not been observed by all the groups,[41,96] and it could be related to the small number of patients in each series. It has been justified, however, with the hypothesis that with a combined modality approach, complete resection becomes not crucial, because the goal of complete tumoral clearance is achieved by the whole treatment. Also, postoperative radiotherapy on a small residual mass may be more effective after induction and in concurrence with adjuvant chemotherapy, allowing a complete clearance of the bed of the tumor.

Masaoka stage 4A tumors enclose patients who have advanced metastatic disease with pleural or pericardial dissemination without distant hematogenous and lymphatic spreading; this category offers a particularly difficult challenge. Although from the oncological point of view this situation represents a disseminated disease, the potential for complete resection should be considered. There are only a few studies reporting management of thymoma at this stage; they are often difficult to interpret, because they span many decades and in many series stages 4A and 4B

are associated. Recently, extended operations like pleurectomy and extrapleural pneumonectomy have been reported with good results.[65,66] Most of the recent cases have been enrolled in a multimodality protocol with induction chemotherapy with a platinum-based regimen (PAC, CAV, VIP) and consolidation therapy after surgery (chemotherapy, radiotherapy, brachytherapy). This combined approach showed increased survival up to 78% at 5 years and 65% at 10 years.[66] Also in this group of patients, preoperative radiotherapy tends to be avoided because of the possibility of increasing the rate of postoperative cardiac complications. There is only one study reporting induction therapy with both chemotherapy and radiation at this stage.[97] Thymic tumors are sensitive to both these means of treatment; thus, it is reasonable to expect a higher complete response rate with this combined approach. This combination modality treatment, however, could limit outcome in many different ways; in fact, dose delivered, toxicity, and surgical morbidity depend on the type of radiation therapy.

Stage 2 thymoma is an heterogeneous category and poses different problems; this group of lesions varies from tumors with microscopic invasion of the capsule to a macroscopic involvement of the capsule and surrounding mediastinal fat, with adhesions to the mediastinal pleura. This category does not include any difference on the basis of the diameter of the tumor and histology. Probably this is the reason why the current therapeutic indications for stage 2 lesions remain controversial. Surgery is the cornerstone and should allow complete resection in all patients, even if partial resections have been reported.[13,18,93] The current indications for postoperative treatment range from radiation therapy in all patients[29,53] to radiation only in patients who have large tumors (greater than 5 cm in diameter) or with radiographic evidence of invasiveness,[13] or patients who have cortical thymoma, well differentiated thymic carcinoma and thymic carcinoma (WHO type B and C),[10] to no radiation at all in any patient.[57]

This debated strategies are based on the assumption and retrospective evidence that at this stage adjuvant radiotherapy does not offer a clear advantage over surgery alone. A more careful evaluation of the results, however, shows that recurrence, whenever it happens, is more frequent within the pleura.[13] This probably justifies the lack of effectiveness of radiotherapy. The authors have observed approximately a 20% rate of recurrence with no standardized postoperative therapy in stage 2 thymoma; since 1989, the authors' policy included postoperative chemoradiotherapy for stage 2B lesions, for tumors with

B and C histology, and those larger than 5 cm in diameter. This policy dramatically reduced the incidence of recurrence, with no recurrence in B WHO type in the following period of time (1989 to 2007, unpublished data). The lack of recurrence also within the mediastinum could be justified by the enhancement of local effect of radiotherapy caused by concomitant administration of chemotherapy.

SUMMARY

Combined modality therapy is gaining acceptance for treating stage 3 and 4A thymic tumors. Also, specific subsets of stage 2 tumors deserve particular attention. Single-center experiences demonstrate that there are some advantages in selected groups of patients. The overall relatively low complete response rate, however, imposes the search for better systemic therapy to optimize results. In fact, although thymic tumors are responsive to different cytotoxic regimens, none has been demonstrated to be the ideal one. New therapies and strategies should be designed and tested in large-scale multicenter prospective trials. Among the others, epidermal growth factor receptor inhibitors have shown some clinical response, because EGFR is overexpressed in thymoma.[98–100] c-KIT[101–103] is overexpressed in thymic carcinoma. Although in a recent study a clinical response to imatinib has been reported, results of a prospective study in patients who have thymic carcinoma are pending.[104] Clinical responses have been reported also to other tyrosine kinase inhibitors, such as dasatinib.[104] Other reports have stressed the presence of an up-regulation of COX-2 with a potential separate therapeutic pathway.[105] Other markers, such as the expression of thymidine synthase and dihydropyrimidine dehydrogenase, which predict sensitivity to 5-fluoruracil-based chemotherapy, were not correlated with the clinicopathological characteristics in a series of thymomas.[106]

These new therapies should be incorporated in a standardized approach that goes from a careful assessment of histology, staging, and lymph node status, and a constructive and nonempiric cooperation between the oncologist, radiotherapist, pathologist, and thoracic surgeon.

REFERENCES

1. Schmidt-Wolf IG, Rockstroh JK, Schuller H, et al. Malignant thymoma: current status of classification and multimodality treatment. Ann Hematol 2003;82:69–76.
2. Detterbeck FC, Parsons AM. Thymic tumors. Ann Thorac Surg 2004;77:1860–9.
3. Gripp S, Hilgers K, Wurm R, et al. Thymoma: prognostic factors and treatment outcome. Cancer 1998;83:1495–503.
4. Detterbeck FC, Parsons AD. Thymic tumors: a review of current diagnosis, classification, and treatment. In: Patterson GA, Cooper JD, Deslauriers J, editors. Pearson's thoracic and esophageal surgery. 3rd edition. Philadelphia: Churchill Livingstone–Elsevier; 2008. p. 1589–614.
5. Wright CD, Wain JC, Wong DR, et al. Predictors of recurrence in thymic tumors: importance of invasion, World Health Organization histology, and size. J Thorac Cardiovasc Surg 2005;130:1413–21.
6. Lopez-Cano M, Ponseti-Bosh JM, Espin-Bosany E, et al. Clinical and pathologic predictors of outcome in thymoma-associated myasthenia gravis. Ann Thorac Surg 2003;76:1643–9.
7. Marino M, Muller-Hermelink HK. Thymoma and thymic carcinoma. Relation of thymoma epithelial cells to the cortical and medullary differentiation of thymus. Virchows Arch 1985;407:119–49.
8. Kirchner T, Marino M, Muller-Hermelink HK. New approaches to the diagnosis of thymic epithelial tumors. Prog Surg Pathol 1989;10:167–89.
9. Pescarmona E, Rendina EA, Venuta F, et al. The prognostic implication of thymoma histologic subtyping. A study of 80 consecutive cases. Am J Clin Pathol 1990;93:190–5.
10. Quintanilla-Martinez L, Wilkins EW Jr, Choi N, et al. Thymoma: histologic classification is an independent prognostic factor. Cancer 1994;74:606–17.
11. Detterbeck FC. Clinical value of the WHO classification system of thymoma. Ann Thorac Surg 2006;81:2328–34.
12. Muller-Hermelink HK, Strobel P, Zetti A, et al. Combined thymic epithelial tumors. In: Travis WD, Brambilla E, Muller-Hermelink HK, editors. Pathology and genetics: tumors of the lung, pleura, thymus, and heart (WHO classification of tumors). Lyon, France: IARC Press; 2004. p. 196–201.
13. Blumberg D, Port JL, Wechsler B, et al. Thymoma: a multivariate analysis of factors predicting survival. Ann Thorac Surg 1995;60:908–14.
14. Kondo K, Monden Y. Therapy of thymic epithelial tumors: a clinical study of 1320 patients from Japan. Ann Thorac Surg 2003;75:878–85.
15. Masaoka A, Monden Y, Nakahara K, et al. Follow-up study of thymomas with special reference to their clinical stages. Cancer 1981;48:2485–92.
16. Nagakawa K, Asamura H, Matsumo Y, et al. Thymoma: a clinicopathological study based on a new World Health Organization classification. J Thorac Cardiovasc Surg 2003;126:1134–40.
17. Masaoka A, Yamakawa Y, Niwa H, et al. Thymectomy and malignancy. Eur J Cardiothorac Surg 1994;8:251–3.
18. Gamondes JP, Balawi A, Greenland T, et al. Seventeen years of surgical treatment of thymoma: factors

influencing survival. Eur J Cardiothorac Surg 1991;5: 124–31.

19. Yamakawa Y, Masaoka A, Hashimoto T, et al. A tentative tumor—node metastasis classification of thymoma. Cancer 1991;68:1984–7.

20. International Union Against Cancer. TNM supplement. A commentary on uniform use,. 3rd edition. New York: Wiley-Liss; 2003.

21. Koga K, Matsuno Y, Noguchi M, et al. A review of 79 thymomas: modification of staging system and reappraisal of conventional division into invasive and non invasive thymoma. Pathol Int 1994;44: 359–67.

22. Verley JM, Hallman KH. Thymoma: a comparative study of clinical stages, histologic features, and survival in 200 cases. Cancer 1985;55:1074–86.

23. Regnard JF, Magdeleinat P, Dromer C, et al. Prognostic factors and long-term results after thymoma resection: a series of 307 patients. J Thorac Cardiovasc Surg 1996;112:376–84.

24. Maggi G, Casadio C, Cavallo A, et al. Thymoma: results of 241 operated cases. Ann Thorac Surg 1991;51:152–6.

25. Ruffini E, Mancuso M, Oliaro A, et al. Recurrence of thymoma: analysis of clinicopathological features, treatment, and outcome. J Thorac Cardiovasc Surg 1997;113:55–63.

26. Okumura M, Ohta M, Tateyama H, et al. The World Health Organization histologic classification system reflects the oncologic behaviour of thymoma: a clinical study of 273 patients. Cancer 2002;94: 624–32.

27. Lewis JE, Wick HR, Scheithauer BW, et al. Thymoma: a clinicopathologic review. Cancer 1987;60: 2727–43.

28. Okumura M, Miyoshi S, Takeuchi Y, et al. Results of surgical treatment of thymomas with special reference to the involved organs. J Thorac Cardiovasc Surg 1999;117:605–13.

29. Nakahara K, Ohno K, Hashimoto J, et al. Thymoma: results with complete resection and adjuvant postoperative irradiation in 141 consecutive patients. J Thorac Cardiovasc Surg 1988;95:1041–7.

30. Monden Y, Nakahara K, Liota S, et al. Recurrent thymoma: clinicopathological features, therapy, and prognosis. Ann Thorac Surg 1985;39:165–9.

31. Wilkins KB, Sheikh E, Green R, et al. Clinical and pathologic predictors of survival in patients with thymoma. Ann Thorac Surg 1999;230:562–74.

32. Pescarmona E, Rendina EA, Venuta F, et al. Analysis of prognostic factors and clinicopathological staging of thymoma. Ann Thorac Surg 1990;50:534–8.

33. Strobel P, Bauer A, Puppe B, et al. Tumor recurrence and survival in patients treated for thymomas and thymic squamous cell carcinomas: a retrospective analysis. J Clin Oncol 2004;22:1501–9.

34. Pan CC, Wun HP, Yang CF, et al. The clinicopathological correlation of epithelial subtyping in thymoma: a study of 112 consecutive cases. Hum Pathol 1994;25:893–9.

35. Chalabreysse L, Roy P, Cordier JF, et al. Correlation of the WHO schema for the classification of thymic neoplasms with prognosis. Am J Surg Pathol 2002; 26:1605–11.

36. Dawson A, Ibrahim NBN, Gibbs AR. Observer variation in histopathological classification of thymoma: correlation with prognosis. Clin Pathol 1994;47:519–23.

37. Lardenois D, Rechsteiner R, Lang RH, et al. Prognostic relevance of Masaoka and Muller–Hermelink classification in patients with thymic tumors. Ann Thorac Surg 2000;69:1550–5.

38. Kondo K, Yoshizawa K, Tsuyuguchi M, et al. WHO histologic classification is a prognostic indicator in thymoma. Ann Thorac Surg 2004;77:1183–8.

39. Park MS, Chung KY, Kim KD, et al. Prognosis of thymic epithelial tumors according to the new World Health Organization histologic classification. Ann Thorac Surg 2004;78:992–7.

40. Chen G, Marx A, Wen-Hu C, et al. New WHO histologic classification predicts prognosis of thymic epithelial tumors: a clinicopathologic study of 200 thymoma cases from China. Cancer 2002;95: 420–9.

41. Venuta F, Rendina EA, Pescarmona E, et al. Multimodality treatment of thymoma: a prospective study. Ann Thorac Surg 1997;64:1585–92.

42. Venuta F, Rendina EA, Longo F, et al. Long-term outcome after multimodality treatment for stage III thymic tumors. Ann Thorac Surg 2003;76:1866–72.

43. Jackson MA, Ball DL. Postoperative radiotherapy in invasive thymoma. Radiother Oncol 1991;21:77–82.

44. Cowen D, Richaud P, Mornex F, et al. Thymoma: results of a multicentric retrospective series of 149 non metastatic irradiated patients and review of the literature. FNCLCC trialists. Federation Nationale des centres de lutte contre le cancer. Radiother Oncol 1995;34:9–16.

45. Wilkins EJ, Edmunds LH, Castleman B. Cases of thymoma at the Massachusetts General Hospital. J Thorac Cardiovasc Surg 1966;52:322–30.

46. Moore KH, Mc Kenzie PR, Kennedy CW, et al. Thymoma: trends over time. Ann Thorac Surg 2001;72:203–7.

47. Kondo K, Monden Y. Thymoma and myasthenia gravis: a clinical study. Ann Thorac Surg 2005;79: 219–24.

48. Wang LS, Huang HH, Lin TS, et al. Malignant thymoma. Cancer 1992;70:443–50.

49. Elert O, Buchwald J, Wolf J. Epithelial thymic tumors—therapy and prognosis. Thorac Cardiovasc Surg 1988;36:109–13.

50. Kondo K, Monden Y. Lymphogenous and hematogenous metastasis of thymic epithelial tumors. Ann Thorac Surg 2003;76:1859–65.

51. Rea F, Marulli G, Girardi R, et al. Long-term survival and prognostic factors in thymic epithelial tumors. Eur J Cardiothorac Surg 2004;26:412–8.

52. Crucitti F, Doglietto GB, Bellantone R, et al. Effects of surgical treatment in thymoma with myasthenia gravis: our experience with 103 patients. J Surg Oncol 1992;50:43–6.

53. Wilkins EJ, Grillo HC, Scannell JG, et al. Role of staging in prognosis and management of thymoma. Ann Thorac Surg 1991;51:888–92.

54. Uematsu M, Kondo M. A proposal for treatment of invasive thymoma. Cancer 1986;58:1979–84.

55. Ariaratnam LS, Kalmiki S, Mincer F, et al. The management of malignant thymoma with radiation therapy. Int J Radiat Oncol Biol Phys 1979;5:77–80.

56. Arrigada R, Marchant-Gerard R, Tribiana M, et al. Radiation therapy in the management of thymic tumors. Acta Radiol Oncol 1981;20:167–72.

57. Singhal S, Shrager JB, Rosenthal DI, et al. Comparison of stages I–II thymoma treated by complete resection with or without adjuvant radiation. Ann Thorac Surg 2003;76:1635–42.

58. Haniuda M, Miyazawa M, Yoshida K, et al. Is postoperative radiotherapy for thymic carcinoma effective? Ann Surg 1996;224:219–24.

59. Akaogi E, Ohara K, Mitsui K, et al. Preoperative radiotherapy and surgery for advanced thymoma with invasion of the great vessels. J Surg Oncol 1996;63:17–22.

60. Urgesi A, Monetti U, Rossi G, et al. Aggressive treatment of intrathoracic recurrences in thymoma. Radiother Oncol 1992;24:221–5.

61. Truong LD, Mody DR, Cagle PT. Thymic carcinoma: a clinicopathologic study of 13 cases. Am J Surg Pathol 1990;14:151–66.

62. Yagi K, Hirata T, Fukuse T, et al. Surgical treatment for invasive thymoma, especially when the superior vena cava is invaded. Ann Thorac Surg 1996;61:521–44.

63. Ogawa K, Uno T, Toita T, et al. Postoperative radiotherapy for patients with completely resected thymoma. Cancer 2002;94:1405–13.

64. Thomas CR, Wright CD, Loherer J. Thymoma: state of the art. J Clin Oncol 1999;17:2280–9.

65. Wright CD. Pleuropneumonectomy for the treatment of Masaoka stage IVA thymoma. Ann Thorac Surg 2006;82:1234–9.

66. Huang J, Rizk NP, Travis WD, et al. Feasibility of multimodality therapy including extended resections in stage IVA thymoma. J Thorac Cardiovasc Surg 2007;134:1477–84.

67. Boston B. Chemotherapy of invasive thymoma. Cancer 1976;38:49–52.

68. Giaccone G. Treatment of malignant thymoma. Curr Opin Oncol 2005;17:140–6.

69. Hu E, Levine J. Chemotherapy of malignant thymoma: case report and review of the literature. Cancer 1986;57:1101–4.

70. Godel N, Boning L, Fredrick A, et al. Chemotherapy of invasive thymoma: a retrospective study of 22 cases. Cancer 1989;63:1493–500.

71. Butler WM, Diehl LF, Taylor HG, et al. Metastatic thymoma with myasthenia gravis. Complete remission with combination chemotherapy. Cancer 1982;50:419–22.

72. Kosmidis PA, Iliopulos E, Penetea S. Combination chemotherapy with cyclophosphamide, adriamycin, and vincristine in malignant thymoma and myasthenia gravis. Cancer 1988;61:1736–40.

73. Dangaard G, Hansen HH, Roth M. Combination chemotherapy for malignant thymoma. Ann Intern Med 1983;99:189–90.

74. Hernandez-Ilizaliturri FJ, Tan D, Cipolla D, et al. Multimodality therapy for thymic carcinoma (TCA): results of a 30-year single institution experience. Am J Clin Oncol 2004;27:68–72.

75. Chalabreysse L, Etienne-Mastroianni B, Adeline P, et al. Thymic carcinoma: a clinicopathological and immunohistological study of 19 cases. Histopathology 2004;44:367–74.

76. De Bree E, van Ruth S, Baas P, et al. Cytoreductive surgery and intraoperative hyperthermic intrathoracic chemotherapy in patients with malignant pleural mesothelioma or pleural metastases of thymoma. Chest 2002;121:1480–7.

77. PJ sr Loehrer, Chen M, Kim K, et al. Cisplatin, doxorubicin, and cyclophosphamide plus thoracic radiation therapy for limited-stage unresectable thymoma: an intergroup trial. J Clin Oncol 1997;15:3093–9.

78. Ohara K, Tatsuraki H, Fuji H, et al. Radioresponse of thymomas verified with histologic response. Acta Oncol 1998;37:471–4.

79. WJ jr Curran, Kornstein MJ, Brooks JJ, et al. Invasive thymoma: the role of mediastinal irradiation following complete or incomplete surgical resection. J Clin Oncol 1988;6:1722–7.

80. Mc Cart JA, Gaspar L, Inculet R, et al. Predictors of survival following surgical resection of thymoma. J Surg Oncol 1993;54:233–8.

81. Pollack A, Komaki R, Cox JC, et al. Thymoma: treatment and prognosis. Int J Radiot Oncol Biol Phys 1992;23:1037–43.

82. Koh WJ, Loehrer PJ Sr, Thomas CR Jr. Thymoma: the role of radiation and chemotherapy. In: Wood DE, Thomas CR, editors. Mediastinal tumors: update 1005. Medical radiology—diagnostic imaging and radiation oncology volume. Heidelberg, Germany: Springer-Verlag; 1995. p. 19–25.

83. Arakawa A, Yesunga T, Sartoh H, et al. Radiation therapy of invasive thymoma. Int J Radiat Oncol Biol Phys 1990;18:529–34.

84. Shin DM, Walsh GL, Kornaki R, et al. A multidisciplinary approach to therapy for unresectable malignant thymoma. Ann Intern Med 1998;204:859–64.

85. Latz D, Schraube P, Oppitz U, et al. Invasive thymoma: treatment with postoperative radiation therapy. Radiology 1997;204:859–64.

86. Mornex F, Rosbeut M, Richard P, et al. Radiotherapy and chemotherapy for invasive thymomas: a multicentric retrospective review of 90 cases. Int Radiat Oncol Biol Phys 1995;32:651–9.

87. Ciernik IF, Meier U, Lutolf VM. Prognostic factors and outcome of incompletely resected invasive thymoma following radiation therapy. J Clin Oncol 1994;12:1484–90.

88. Kundel J, Yellin A, Popovitzer A, et al. Adjuvant radiotherapy for thymic epithelial tumors. Treatment results and prognostic factors. Am J Clin Oncol 2007;30:389–94.

89. Ichinose Y, Ohta M, Yano T, et al. Treatment of invasive thymoma with pleural dissemination. J Surg Oncol 1993;54:180.

90. Myojin M, Choi NC, Wright CD, et al. Stage III thymoma: patterns of failure after surgery and postoperative radiotherapy and its implications for future stuffy. Int J Radiat Oncol Biol Phys 2000;46:927–33.

91. Rea F, Sartori F, Loy M, et al. Chemotherapy and operation for invasive thymoma. J Thorac Cardiovasc Surg 1993;106:543–9.

92. Lucchi M, Ambrogi MC, Duranti L, et al. Advanced-stage thymomas and thymic carcinomas: results of multimodality treatment. Ann Thorac Surg 2005;79:1840–4.

93. Macchiarini P, Chella A, Ducci F, et al. Neoadjuvant chemotherapy, surgery and postoperative radiation therapy for invasive thymoma. Cancer 1991;68:706–13.

94. Ribet M, Voisin C, Pruvot FR, et al. Lympho-epithelial thymomas: a retrospective study of 88 resections. Eur J Cardiothorac Surg 1988;2:261–4.

95. Gewrychowski J, Rockicki M, Gabriel A, et al. Thymoma—the usefulness of some prognostic factors for diagnosis and surgical treatment. Eur J Surg Oncol 2000;26:203–8.

96. Kim ES, Putnam JB, Komaki R, et al. Phase II study of a multidisciplinary approach with induction chemotherapy followed by surgical resection, radiation therapy, and consolidation chemotherapy for unresectable malignant thymomas: final report. Lung Cancer 2004;44:369–79.

97. Wright CD, Noah CC, Wain JC, et al. Induction chemoradiotherapy followed by resection for locally advanced Masaoka stage III and IVA thymic tumors. Ann Thorac Surg 2008;85:385–9.

98. Hanley JD, Koukolis GH, Loehrer PJ, et al. Epidermal growth factor expression in invasive thymoma. J Cancer Res Clin Oncol 2002;128:167–70.

99. Palmieri G, Marino M, Salvatore M, et al. Cetuximab is an active treatment of metastatic and chemorefractory thymoma. Front Biosci 2007;12:167–70.

100. Yamaguchi H, Sada H, Kitezoki T, et al. Thymic carcinoma with epidermal growth factor receptor gene mutations. Lung Cancer 2006;52:261–2.

101. Henley JD, Cummings OW, Loehrer PJ sr. Tyrosine kinase receptor expression in thymomas. J Cancer Res Oncol 2004;130:222–4.

102. Pan CC, Chen PCH, Chiang H. KIT (CD117) is frequently overexpressed in thymic carcinomas but is absent in thymomas. J Pathol 2004;202:375–81.

103. Nakagawa K, Matsuno Y, Kumitoh H, et al. Immunohistochemical KIT (CD117) expression in thymic epithelial tumors. Chest 2005;128:140–4.

104. Strobel P, Hartman M, Jakob A, et al. Thymic carcinoma with overexpression of mutated KIT and the response to Imatinib. N Engl J Med 2004;350:2625–6.

105. Rickter RJ, Joos S, Mechtersheimer G, et al. COX-2 up-regulation in thymomas and thymic carcinomas. Int J Cancer 2006;119:2063–70.

106. Sasaki H, Fukai I, Kiriyama M, et al. Thymidilate synthase and dihydropyrimidine dehydrogenase mRNA levels in thymoma. Surg Today 2003;33:83–8.

Surgical Approaches to the Thymus in Patients with Myasthenia Gravis

Mitchell J. Magee, MD, Michael J. Mack, MD*

KEYWORDS

- Myasthenia gravis • Surgery • Thymectomy
- Thymus gland • Thoracoscopy • VATS

Myasthenia gravis (MG) is an autoimmune disorder of neuromuscular transmission affecting 2 out of every 100,000 people. In 1939, Blalock[1] reported remission of generalized MG following removal of a cystic thymic tumor in a 21-year-old woman. Subsequently, Blalock and colleagues[2,3] reported improvement in at least half of the patients with MG in whom they performed thymectomy and found hyperplasia in the thymus glands without thymoma. Since these reports, thymectomy, with or without the presence of thymoma, has been considered important in the treatment of MG, though neurologists and surgeons still debate what role surgery should play in the management of nonthymomatous MG. Central to this debate is the lack of randomized controlled trials comparing surgery, medical therapy, and the natural history of the disease, and disagreement among surgeons as to what constitutes the best surgical therapy. Further adding to the controversy, until recently,[4,5] has been the lack of universally accepted classifications, grading systems, and methods of analysis for patients undergoing surgical therapy for MG. Most surgeons agree that improved clinical outcomes correlate with completeness of thymectomy and currently the majority of surgeons use the median sternotomy approach, removing primarily the encapsulated thymus with varying extents of adjacent mediastinal fat. Anatomic reports on the common presence of widely distributed ectopic thymic tissue[6–8] coupled with reports of complete responses to excision of residual thymic tissue after failed initial thymectomy have prompted some surgeons to advocate a more extensive cervical and transsternal mediastinal dissection aimed at more complete removal of all thymic tissue. Other surgeons favor less invasive approaches to thymectomy, citing similar response rates with less radical removal of thymic associated tissue.

As summarized in the recommendations for clinical research standards in myasthenia gravis,[4,5] the debate is not resolved regarding which of the multiple techniques that have been described for removal of the thymus in MG is ideal. Although, classically, total thymectomy is considered the goal of surgery, it has not been demonstrated unequivocally that this is necessary, nor is it clear that all the resectional techniques do achieve this goal. The Myasthenia Gravis Foundation of America (MGFA) Thymectomy Classification was proposed in an attempt to apply objectivity and consistency in reporting of the various approaches and techniques employed when removing thymus tissue in patients with myasthenia gravis (**Box 1**).

In this article the authors describe the various surgical approaches to the thymus currently used in the management of patients with nonthymomatous MG, incorporating the MGFA Classification scheme, and demonstrate the rationale, limitations, and published data supporting the use of each of these approaches.

TRANSCERVICAL THYMECTOMY

The transcervical approach was first described and proposed as a suitable alternative for thymectomy in patients with MG by Crile[9] and subsequently substantiated by Kirschner and colleagues.[10,11] This basic transcervical

Cardiopulmonary Research Science Technology Institute, 7777 Forest Lane, Suite A-323, Dallas, TX 75230, USA
* Corresponding author.
E-mail address: mmack@csant.com (M.J. Mack).

Thorac Surg Clin 19 (2009) 83–89
doi:10.1016/j.thorsurg.2008.09.013
1547-4127/08/$ – see front matter © 2009 Elsevier Inc. All rights reserved.

thymectomy, as it was initially employed, is now universally considered inadequate and has been abandoned. The accepted technique now defined as extended transcervical thymectomy, described and popularized by Cooper,[12] has been used successfully with reports of satisfactory results by several groups.[12–15] The patient is placed supine with an inflatable bag placed behind the shoulders to allow hyperextension of the neck. A 4 cm incision is placed in a skin crease at the base of the neck with the midpoint positioned 2 cm above the sternal notch. The subplatysmal plane is developed caudally down to the sternum and cephalad to the inferior border of the thyroid gland. The ligamentous insertions of the sternocleidomastoid muscles are divided vertically to expose and enter the substernal plane. The strap muscles are separated in the midline and the upper poles of the thymus gland are identified behind the strap muscles. The upper poles are individually dissected free, down to their union just above the sternal notch, and the dissection continued down to the innominate vein. The plane between the thymus and the sternum is created with blunt digital dissection to allow placement of the Cooper Thymectomy Retractor (Pilling Co., Fort Washington, Pennsylvania). The sternum is retracted anteriorly, completely suspending the chest by the manubrium, as the shoulder bag is deflated and the neck and upper back maximally extended. Two Parker retractors are placed in the upper corners of the incision and fixed to the table to provide countertraction. The surgeon is seated at the head of the bed with a headlight. The upper poles of the thymus are gently retracted anterior and cephalad by silk ligatures, exposing the venous drainage of

the thymus into the innominate vein (**Fig. 1**). These veins are divided between silk ligatures. The dissection is then continued bluntly posteriorly between the thymus and pericardium into the mediastinum with a Kitner dissector. Small branches between the thymus and the internal mammary artery may be encountered from the left or right and are divided with electrocautery, taking care to avoid injury to the phrenic nerves. In most cases the completely encapsulated thymus gland is removed intact with both upper poles and both lower poles in continuity.[12,15,16] No drains are required. Proponents of the transcervical approach cite similar remission rates with less morbidity and shorter mean length of hospital stay when compared with transsternal approaches. Limitations of the transcervical approach include: (1) a comparatively less radical resection of thymic tissue is conceptually less desirable and, though debatable, may be associated with poorer outcomes; (2) the unique nature of this approach makes it difficult to teach, learn, and consistently reproduce and, therefore, has limited adoption; and (3) the neck incision may not be considered as cosmetically acceptable.

VIDEOTHORACOSCOPIC THYMECTOMY

The classic video-assisted thoracoscopic surgery (VATS) thymectomy is our preferred approach and has several permutations including left-side, right-side, bilateral, and subxyphoid. In the

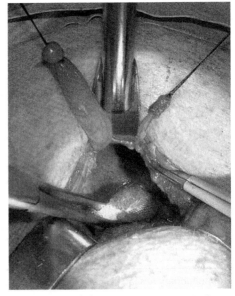

Fig. 1. Transcervical thymectomy: surgeon's view with Cooper Thymectomy Retractor in place and the upper poles of the thymus retracted by silk ligatures.

majority of cases the authors favor a unilateral right-sided approach. The patient is positioned in a 30° partial lateral, with a roll behind the right scapula, the left arm tucked along the patient's side, and the right arm elevated on an arm board. The first of three 5 mm trocars is placed at the apex of an inverted triangle positioned half-way between the xyphoid and the sternal notch, in the posterior axillary line. A 5mm 30° video-thoracoscope is placed through this trocar, and after confirming collapse of the right lung, two additional 5 mm trocars are placed under direct vision. Both of these trocars are placed in the midaxillary line, with one placed two interspaces caudal and the other two interspaces cephalad to the camera port, and provide working channels for instruments (**Fig. 2**). The assistant holds the camera, standing on the same side of the table and to the right of the surgeon, and elevates the thymic tissue using a fan retractor placed through a 10–12 mm port. This last port is placed later in the procedure and positioned caudal and anterior to the other ports, in either the midaxillary or anterior axillary line. This incision will also be used for specimen retrieval after completion of the thymectomy. The 30° scope is essential in providing adequate visualization of the cervical region, cephalad to the innominate vein, and left posterolateral extents of the dissection approaching the left phrenic nerve. With minimal trauma produced by the 5 mm trocars, we have not hesitated to add or replace a trocar as needed to facilitate the dissection.

High-flow carbon dioxide insufflation is routinely used with pressure limits set at 8 mm Hg. This greatly facilitates: (1) collapse of the right lung, (2) access to and dissection of the mediastinal tissue planes, and (3) enhanced visualization of the cephalad extent of the cervical dissection. Routine instrumentation in addition to the videothoracoscope and trocars includes: 5 mm endoscopic graspers or Debakey forceps, 5 mm hook electrocautery instrument, 5 mm ultrasonic harmonic scalpel, 5 mm endoscopic Kittner dissectors, 5 mm medium endoscopic hemoclip appliers, and a 10 mm endoscopic fan retractor.

The unilateral right-sided approach is preferred because of relative increased working space absent the left ventricle, and the superior vena cava serves as an excellent landmark for initial dissection and identification of the innominate vein. We first identify important anatomic landmarks including the superior vena cava, right phrenic nerve, right internal mammary vessels, and the thymus within surrounding mediastinal fat.

The dissection is begun caudally, scoring the mediastinal pleura just anterior to the right phrenic nerve, and continued cephalad to the junction of the superior vena cava and innominate vein. The hook cautery set at 25–30 W is expeditious and works well for much of this dissection. Recently, we have used the ultrasonic harmonic shears which work equally well closed as a blunt dissector, provide better hemostasis of larger vessels, produce less plume, and are less likely to injure surrounding structures with conduction of heat and electric current. The dissection is continued anteriorly behind the right internal mammary vessels, along the posterior sternum toward the left, and then back caudally and posterior to the pericardial reflection, returning to the initial point of dissection. The posterior portion of the dissection is completed first in the avascular plain between the thymus and pericardium. All anterior mediastinal tissue is included and removed off of the pericardium and superior vena cava up to the innominate vein, and then similarly dissected off of the sternum by gentle posterior retraction, taking care to bluntly sweep the left pleural attachments off of the mediastinal tissues. Then, beginning at the superior vena caval innominate vein junction, the dissection continues along the caudal border of the innominate vein where the arterial supply and venous drainage is usually encountered. The fan retractor facilitates exposure by retracting thymic tissue caudal and laterally toward the patient's left. The thymic vessels are clipped using an endoscopic clip applier and or divided with the ultrasonic harmonic shears. Division of the thymic venous drainage significantly improves exposure and dissection posterior to the innominate vein. Devascularization of the thymus allows easier discrimination of the deeper yellow thymic tissue from adjacent mediastinal fat.

The cervical dissection of the superior poles of the thymus is performed next. Excellent visualization is achieved by proper positioning and

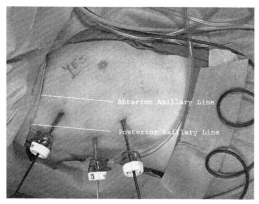

Fig. 2. VATS thymectomy: right-sided approach, initial port placement.

angulation of the 30° scope. Gentle caudal traction using the endoscopic grasper alternating with the ultrasonic shears functioning as an endoscopic grasper, blunt dissector, and sharp dissector with cauterization, separates the ligamentous attachments from the superior poles of the thymus. The right superior pole is dissected and teased completely out of the neck followed by the left superior pole dissected similarly.

The final and most technically challenging step in the dissection is the left lateral posterior separation of thymic tissue from the left pleural and pericardial attachments approaching the left phrenic nerve. This dissection may begin wherever it is easiest, but most often is begun cephalad near the junction of the innominate vein and left internal mammary vessels and progresses caudal and posterior toward the pericardial phrenic recess. Although the left phrenic nerve can be visualized in many cases, no concerted effort is made to specifically do so, but constant vigilance is maintained to identify the nerve and avoid injury if it is encountered. Accordingly, the majority of this dissection is done bluntly, retracting the thymic tissue and adjacent fat caudal and to the right with the fan retractor, and sweeping the left pleura veil to the left. Repositioning the fan to retract tissue more anteriorly and to the right and rotating the operating table to the right, thereby allowing gravity to facilitate retraction, the tissue between the left phrenic nerve and pericardium can be safely and completely removed. We try to maintain integrity of the left pleura as it makes the exposure easier, but the left pleural space is often entered and is usually of no consequence.

Once the entire specimen is free of surrounding attachments, it is placed in an endoscopic bag placed through the 10–12 mm trocar used previously for the fan retractor. This trocar incision will occasionally require minimal enlargement to deliver larger specimens. The resected specimen is examined for completeness of resection and the anterior mediastinum is then reinspected for any residual thymic tissue and for hemostasis. Irrigation fluid collected in the right chest is removed, and a pediatric feeding tube is placed through the cephalad anterior trocar site and placed under water seal to evacuate air from the chest cavities as the lung is reexpanded. Drains are not routinely placed unless there is suspected lung injury. Tomulescu and colleagues[17] compared the right- and left-sided approaches to VATS thymectomy and found similar operating times, length of hospitalization, and rates of remission. No differences in operative complications were noted. In their experience, the left-side approach is preferred due to the majority of mediastinal fat being located on the left side of the anterior mediastinum, making dissection of the thymus on the contralateral side safer and easier. They further believe that the risk of injury to the right phrenic nerve is decreased due to its location outside the surgical field and that the left side affords needed access to the aortopulmonary window. Several centers including our own have reported intermediate-term MG remission rates comparable to more invasive approaches to thymectomy.[18–20] Cited advantages of the VATS approach include decreased blood loss, decreased length of hospital stay, improved cosmetic result, faster recovery and social reintegration, and less pain. As opposed to the skills needed to obtain the unique exposure required for transcervical thymectomy, a VATS thymectomy can be easily learned and performed safely and effectively by most thoracic surgeons experienced in advanced videothoracoscopy. Similar to the transcervical approach, VATS achieves a less radical resection of thymic tissue which debatably is less desirable because of the potential for poorer outcomes.

The authors recently retrospectively reviewed their experience in 48 patients with myasthenia gravis, who underwent VATS thymectomy between March 1992 and June 2006. Patients were assessed using MGFA guidelines with clinical visits or by telephone interview and follow-up was greater than 90%; complete with a mean postoperative period of follow-up of 6 years. Mean hospital postoperative length of stay was 1.9 days. Complete stable remission was seen in 34.9%, minimal manifestations seen in an additional 55.8%, and two patients (4%) were worse postoperatively. These results were similar to those observed in a comparable group of 47 MG patients who underwent extended transsternal thymectomy during the same time period.

Mantegazza[21] published a follow-up report on a technique described by Novellino[22] as VATET, consisting of bilateral thoracoscopy and open cervical exploration. VATET essentially combines elements of the VATS and transcervical approaches to achieve a more thorough extirpation of thymic tissue. Two hundred and six MG patients underwent either the VATET or extended transsternal thymectomy, and were followed for 6 years. The 159 patients that underwent the VATET procedure had comparable complete stable remission rates to the 47 patients that had an extended transsternal thymectomy (50.6% versus 48.7%).[23] Shigemura and colleagues[24] prospectively studied the contribution of the transcervical exploration to the VATET procedure and concluded that additional thymus tissue can be removed through a cervical incision following bilateral VATS thymectomy, although the clinical significance of this has not been demonstrated.

ROBOTIC-ASSISTED THYMECTOMY

The incorporation of complete robotic surgical systems, such as the da Vinci (Intuitive Surgical Inc.), has been proposed by some to enhance precision maneuverability in the mediastinum when compared with conventional VATS thymectomy. Augustin and colleagues[25] recently published a review of the 32 institutional-reported robotic thymectomies, including their own experience, and compared robotic-assisted thoracoscopic surgery (RATS) to VATS thymectomy. The left-sided operative approach is preferred with the robotic endoscope positioned in the midaxillary line sixth intercostal space, and two robotic instrument ports placed in the third and sixth intercostal spaces. While the feasibility and safety of RATS thymectomy with the da Vinci system has been proven, the benefits of, or value added by, the RATS approach to thymectomy, compared with the conventional VATS approach have not yet been demonstrated. Proponents of robot-assisted thymectomy[25,26] opine that robotic surgery is more suitable than VATS for an extended thymectomy because of easier dissection of the upper horns, more controlled ligation of the thymic veins, and improved unilateral access to the entire anterior mediastinum.

TRANSSTERNAL THYMECTOMY

Transsternal thymectomy is the most common approach used in the surgical treatment of MG. The basic transsternal thymectomy, as it was originally performed by Blalock,[1] has been abandoned in favor of more extensive resections that can be easily achieved through the same or a smaller incision; eg, upper partial sternotomy, with similar or less morbidity. Masaoka and colleagues[8] identified thymic tissue in adipose tissue located outside the thymic capsule in the anterior mediastinum in 13 of 18 MG patients undergoing thymectomy. Based on this observation, they recommended removal of all adipose tissue in the anterior mediastinum along with the gross thymus via an extended thymectomy. A detailed description of the procedure along with their 20-year experience was subsequently reported.[27] Following a full sternotomy, an en bloc resection of the thymus gland and all anterior mediastinal adipose tissue is completed, including all adipose tissue around the upper poles of the thymus, the brachiocephalic vein, and the pericardium. The borders of resection are the diaphragm caudally, the thyroid gland cephalad, and the phrenic nerves bilaterally (**Fig. 3**). Two hundred

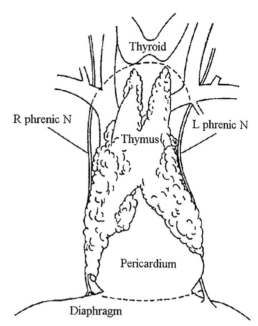

Fig. 3. Transsternal thymectomy: Borders of resection are the diaphragm caudally, the thyroid gland cephalad, and the phrenic nerves bilaterally. L, left; N, nerve; R, right.

and eighty-six patients with nonthymomatous MG underwent extended transsternal thymectomy between 1973 and 1993. Remission rates were 36.9% at 3 years, 45.8% at 5 years, 55.7% at 10 years, and 67.2% at 15 years. Venuta and colleagues[28] reported their experience with 232 thymectomies performed between 1970 and 1997. One hundred and one patients with nonthymomatous MG had an extended thymectomy through a partial upper sternotomy. After a mean postoperative follow-up of 119 months, 25% of the patients were in complete remission and an additional 46% were clinically improved. There were two operative deaths (0.9%) due to respiratory failure in patients with postoperative bleeding requiring reoperation, and seven patients in the nonthymomatous group (4.5%) died from MG (mean survival: 34.3 ± 3.6 months). Minor complications included arrhythmia (1.8%) and infection (1.8%) and mean postoperative hospital stay was 6.4 days. Allowing again for differences in severity of disease and methods of reporting outcomes, the results of extended transsternal thymectomy appear to be comparable to other approaches but associated with significant morbidity.

TRANSCERVICAL AND TRANSSTERNAL THYMECTOMY

The primary proponent and practitioner of the transcervical and transsternal ("maximal") thymectomy approach are Jaretzki and Wolff.[7] Wide exposure in the neck and mediastinum is achieved through a complete median sternotomy incision and separate collar incision. The skin incisions are occasionally connected to create a "T," but the subcutaneous and deeper planes of dissection in the neck and mediastinum are always confluent. All thymus, suspected thymus, and mediastinal fat, including both mediastinal pleural sheets, are removed en bloc using sharp dissection on the pleurae and pericardium. The entire dissection is performed and completed "as if it was an en bloc dissection for a malignant tumor."[29] Starting at the diaphragm, the dissection extends from hilum to hilum and proceeds cephalad to the innominate vein. After elevating the strap muscles above the innominate vein, the cervical dissection is begun and continued posterior to the strap muscles to the level of the thyroid cartilage, removing thymic tissue posterior and superior to the thyroid gland and adjacent to the recurrent laryngeal and vagus nerves. This is certainly conceptually the technique most likely to remove all thymic tissue, but this radical extirpation is associated with the most morbidity and least desirable cosmetic result. Advocates for this approach, believing it the most effective in achieving a durable complete remission, also believe that the end results justify the means. Alternatively, the authors argue that in the absence of controlled prospective clinical trials showing a clear benefit to more radical complete removal of all gross and microscopic thymic tissue, a more balanced approach between procedure-related morbidity and complete thymectomy is warranted.

Many patients with MG who might benefit from thymectomy are denied the opportunity because of misconceptions, ignorance, or trepidation. By offering effective methods of less invasive thymectomy to patients with MG, a significant number of patients and treating neurologists previously unwilling to consider surgery may realize the benefits of this established, proven treatment alternative.

REFERENCES

1. Blalock A, Mason MF, Morgan HJ, et al. Myasthenia gravis and tumors of the thymic region. Report of a case in which the tumor was removed. Ann Surg 1939;110:544–61.
2. Blalock A, Harvey AM, Ford FR, et al. The treatment of myasthenia gravis by removal of the thymus gland. Preliminary report. JAMA 1945;127:1089–96.
3. Blalock A. Thymectomy in the treatment of myasthenia gravis. Report of twenty cases. J Thorac Surg 1944;13:316–39.
4. Jaretzki A III, Barohn RJ, Ernstoff RM, et al. Myasthenia gravis: recommendations for clinical research standards. Neurology 2000;55:16–23.
5. Jaretzki A III, Barohn RJ, Ernstoff RM, et al. Myasthenia gravis: recommendations for clinical research standards. Ann Thorac Surg 2000;70:327–34.
6. Jaretzki A III, Bethea M, Wolff M, et al. A rational approach to total thymectomy in the treatment of myasthenia gravis. Ann Thorac Surg 1977;24(2):120–30.
7. Jaretzki A III, Wolff M. "Maximal" thymectomy for myasthenia gravis: surgical anatomy and operative technique. J Thorac Cardiovasc Surg 1988;96:711–6.
8. Masaoka A, Nagaoka Y, Kotake Y. Distribution of thymic tissue at the anterior mediastinum: current procedures in thymectomy. J Thorac Cardiovasc Surg 1975;70:747–54.
9. Crile G Jr. Thymectomy through the neck. Surgery 1966;59:213–5.
10. Kirschner PA, Osserman KE, Kark AE. Studies in myasthenia gravis: transcervical total thymectomy. JAMA 1969;209:906–10.
11. Kark AE, Kirschner PA. Total thymectomy by the transcervical approach. Br J Surg 1971;58:323–6.
12. Cooper JD, Al-Jilaihawa AN, Pearson FG, et al. An improved technique to facilitate transcervical thymectomy for myasthenia gravis. Ann Thorac Surg 1988;45:242–7.
13. Shrager JB, Deeb ME, Mick R, et al. Transcervical thymectomy for myasthenia gravis achieves results comparable to thymectomy by sternotomy. Ann Thorac Surg 2002;74:320–7.
14. Shrager JB, Nathan D, Brinster CJ, et al. Outcomes after 151 extended transcervical thymectomies for myasthenia gravis. Ann Thorac Surg 2006;82:1863–9.
15. Calhoun RF, Ritter JH, Guthrie TJ, et al. Results of transcervical thymectomy for myasthenia gravis in 100 consecutive patients. Ann Surg 1999;230:555–61.
16. Meyers BF, Cooper JD. Transcervical thymectomy for myasthenia gravis. Available at: www.ctsnet.org/sections/clinicalresources/thoracic/expert_tech-23.html. Accessed November 15, 2008.
17. Tomulescu V, Ion V, Kosa A, et al. Thoracoscopic thymectomy mid-term results. Ann Thorac Surg 2006;82:1003–7.
18. Mack MJ, Landreneau RJ, Yim AP, et al. Results of video-assisted thymectomy in patients with myasthenia gravis. J Thorac Cardiovasc Surg 1996;112:1352–60.
19. Savcenko M, Wendt GK, Prince SL, et al. Video-assisted thymectomy for myasthenia gravis: an update of a single institution experience. Eur J Cardiothorac Surg 2002;22:978–83.
20. Manlulu A, Lee TW, Wan I, et al. Video-assisted thoracic surgery thymectomy for nonthymomatous myasthenia gravis. Chest 2005;128:3454–60.

21. Mantegazza R, Confalonieri P, Antozzi C, et al. Video-assisted thoracoscopic extended thymectomy (VATET) in myasthenia gravis two-year follow-up in 101 patients and comparison with the transsternal approach. Ann N Y Acad Sci 1998;841:749–52.

22. Novellino L, Longoni M, Spinelli L, et al. "Extended" thymectomy, without sternotomy performed by cervicotomy and thoracoscopic technique in the treatment of myasthenia gravis. Int Surg 1994;79:378–81.

23. Mantegazza R, Baggi F, Bernasconi P, et al. Video-assisted thoracoscopic extended thymectomy and extended transsternal thymectomy (T-3b) in non-thymomatous myasthenia gravis patients: remission after 6 years of follow-up. J Neurol Sci 2003;212(1–2):31–6.

24. Shigemura N, Shiono H, Inoue M, et al. Inclusion of the transcervical approach in video-assisted thoracoscopic extended thymectomy (VATET) for myasthenia gravis: a prospective trial. Surg Endosc 2006;20:1614–8.

25. Augustin F, Schmid T, Sieb M, et al. Video-assisted thoracoscopic surgery versus robotic-assisted thoracoscopic surgery thymectomy. Ann Thorac Surg 2008;85:S768–71.

26. Savitt MA, Gao G, Furnary AP, et al. Application of robotic-assisted techniques to the surgical evaluation and treatment of the anterior mediastinum. Ann Thorac Surg 2005;79:450–5 [discussion: 455].

27. Masaoka A, Yamakawa Y, Niwa H, et al. Extended thymectomy for myasthenia gravis patients: a 20-year review. Ann Thorac Surg 1996;62:853–9.

28. Venuta F, Rendina EA, Giacomo TD, et al. Thymectomy for myasthenia gravis: a 27-year experience. Eur J Cardiothorac Surg 1999;15:621–5.

29. Sonett JR, Jaretzki A III. Thymectomy for nonthymomatous myasthenia gravis: a critical analysis. Ann N Y Acad Sci 2008;1132:315–28.

Vascular Lesions of the Mediastinum

Percy Boateng, MD*, Waqas Anjum, MD, Andrew S. Wechsler, MD

KEYWORDS

- Vascular lesions of the mediastinum
- Mediastinal lymphangioma
- Superior venal caval aneurysms
- Azygous vein aneurysms
- Pulmonary artery and vein aneurysm
- Aortic aneurysm
- Bronchial artery aneurysm
- Mediastinal hemangiomas

Vascular lesions of the mediastinum represent only about 10% of all radiographically recognized mediastinal masses.[1,2] Vascular lesions thus are more likely to be mistaken for the more common solid tumors of the mediastinum. Accurate clinical diagnosis of these vascular entities can help avoid unnecessary diagnostic or surgical intervention.

This article highlights the vascular lesions that present as mediastinal masses. Some radiographic findings represent interesting clinical findings that do not require further intervention, such as a persistent left superior vena cava (LSVC). Differentiating these findings from true pathologic entities then becomes paramount. In other cases, the clinical presentation will prompt immediate surgical or medical management to mitigate or prevent the mortality and morbidity associated with the condition, such as acute aortic dissection. Although specific details about the management of each clinical or pathologic entity are beyond the scope of this article, a brief mention is made of currently recommended therapy where appropriate.

The mediastinum classically is described as either a three- or four-compartment model with an anterior, middle, and posterior region common to both models.[3] The four-compartment model distinguishes a superior compartment that is actually a composite of the superior portions of the anterior, middle, and posterior divisions (**Fig. 1**). The middle mediastinum also is referred to as the visceral compartment, and the posterior, as the paravertebral sulcus. Most vascular lesions arise from the visceral compartment. It is important to remember that the divisions of the mediastinum create a convenient way to localize the pathologic entity, and vascular lesions that originate in one compartment can project into another compartment. The location of the mass and knowledge of the contents of that compartment serve as guides to making an educated guess as to the etiology of the mass.

Vascular lesions of the mediastinum have been described and classified by Kelly and colleagues[4] and Shields and colleagues[5] according to the vascular tissue or organ of origin. Using this classification system, vascular lesions are systemic venous, pulmonary arterial, pulmonary venous, or systemic arterial in origin. Vascular lesions of lymphatic origin also are considered in this discussion. Additionally, other classification schemes can be used to describe these lesions. Vascular lesions can be post-traumatic, neoplastic, congenital, or acquired. Some lesions in the pediatric population are associated with congenital heart disease; a few of these lesions remain undiagnosed until adulthood and then present as mediastinal masses.

Most vascular lesions are first noted as incidental masses on radiographs obtained for other reasons. A few lesions present with dramatic

Department of Cardiothoracic Surgery, Drexel University College of Medicine, North Tower, 7th Floor, Suite 744, Philadelphia, PA, USA
* Corresponding author.
E-mail address: percy.boateng@drexelmed.edu (P. Boateng).

Thorac Surg Clin 19 (2009) 91–105
doi:10.1016/j.thorsurg.2008.09.003

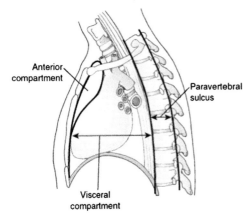

Fig. 1. Three-compartment model. (*From* Raymond DP, Daniel TM. Mediastinal anatomy and mediastinoscopy. In: Selke FW, del Nido PJ, Swanson SJ, editors. Sabiston and Spencer surgery of the chest. 7th edition. Philadelphia: Elsevier Saunders; 2005. p. 668; with permission.)

symptoms (eg, a ruptured aortic aneurysm) or with symptoms caused by the effect of the mass.

The diagnostic methods available for viewing or evaluating masses of the mediastinum include ultrasound/echocardiography, CT scans, MRI, angiography, and fluoroscopy. Before the advent of the current generation of spiral CT scans with angiographic capabilities, MRI is still considered the study of choice for evaluating mediastinal masses suspected to be of vascular origin. A multislice CT scan with multiplanar reconstruction now rivals MRI and is often the only study required to make the diagnosis. MRI remains required when CT scan findings are equivocal or when the patient cannot tolerate iodinated contrast medium. Echocardiography plays a significant role in the neonatal or pediatric population, and echocardiograms are usually sufficient to make the diagnosis. Rarely, angiography and fluoroscopy are used.

LYMPHATIC LESIONS

Lymphangiomas, or cystic hygromas, are benign lesions commonly found in the neck, but they also can be completely intrathoracic (**Fig. 2**)[6] Primary thoracic lymphangiomas are rare lesions and comprise less than 1% of all mediastinal cystic masses.[7] Cases have been documented in patients as young as 5 months and as old as 74 years.[8] They result from abnormal collections of lymph channels that develop early in the embryonic phase.[9] Lymphangiomas grow around normal tissue.[10] They can become extensive and can infiltrate these organs, often preventing complete excision. They can occur in any compartment but frequently are found in the anterior and middle compartments[8] and rarely in the heart.[11] The clinically described subtypes are cavernous lymphangioma and cystic lymphangioma or both combined. These two entities are identical histologically. Lymphangiomas are usually asymptomatic. When symptoms do occur, they are because of the effect of the mass, with a persistent cough sometimes being the only symptom.[9] Other symptoms include infection, hemorrhage, chylothorax, chylopericardium, and superior vena caval syndrome.[8,9,12] On CT scan or MRI images, mediastinal lymphangiomas present as well circumscribed cystic lesions. Several reports indicate that prepathologic diagnosis is difficult, because these lesions are difficult to distinguish from other cystic lesions of the mediastinum.[13,14] Complete surgical excision is recommended when feasible,

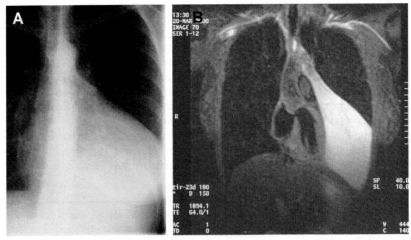

Fig. 2. (*A*) Chest radiograph showing large cystic lymphangioma. (*B*) MRI of the same lesion. (*From* Bossert T, Gummert JF, Mohr FW. Giant cystic lymphangioma of the mediastinum. Eur J Cardiothorac Surg 2002;21(2):340; with permission.)

because incomplete resection almost certainly leads to recurrence. If, however, the mass is extensive or involves vital structures that cannot be sacrificed, then partial resection is acceptable and can result in ameliorated symptoms. Sclerotherapy with OK-432 has shown promising results with unresectable lymphangiomas elsewhere in the body.[15]

THE SYSTEMIC VENOUS SYSTEM

The mediastinal systemic venous system is located in the middle and posterior regions of the mediastinum. Aneurysms and dilatation of the superior vena cava (SVC), innominate vein, and azygous and hemiazygous veins can present as mediastinal masses. A persistent LSVC also can present as a mediastinal mass and occasionally has been misinterpreted as mediastinal adenopathy.[16]

Aneurysmal enlargement of the SVC can be idiopathic (rare), and only a few cases are reported in the literature. Saccular aneurysms as large as 7 cm have been described and successfully treated with surgical resection.[17] Joseph and colleagues[18] reported the association of cystic hygromas and SVC aneurysms.

No clear guidelines exist for when surgical intervention is indicated, and most of the cases reported were operated on to eliminate the risk of complications or because they presented with significant clinical symptoms.

The SVC is dilated more commonly as a result of an increase in central venous pressure caused by tricuspid valvular heart disease, heart failure, or a pericardial process.[5] Other processes such as mediastinal fibrosis, neoplasm, arterial aneurysm, or lymphadenopathy cause either complete or partial obstruction and present as SVC enlargement.[5] On chest radiographs, SVC enlargement or aneurysm presents as a widening of the right side of the mediastinum (**Fig. 3**). Partial anomalous venous return, associated with sinus venous syndrome, also can produce enlargement of the SVC.[4] Typically, the right upper and middle lobe veins, either as a single tributary (superior pulmonary vein) and rarely as separate veins, drain into the SVC or the caval–atrial junction.[19]

A persistent LSVC is reported to occur in 0.5% of normal individuals and in 5% of individuals who have congenital heart disease.[4,20] This finding is associated at a much higher rate with cor triatriatum.[21] The radiographic appearance, which gives the impression of a widened aortic shadow or paramediastinal bulging, results from the persistence of the left anterior and common cardinal veins and left sinus horn.[20,22] Most patients also have a right SVC. The left SVC normally drains into the coronary sinus but can drain into the left atrium, creating a small nonphysiologic right-to-left shunt. It can be associated with an unroofed coronary sinus syndrome. The radiographic appearance of a persistent LSVC has been misinterpreted as mediastinal lymphadenopathy.[16] Cavopulmonary anastomotic aneurysm of the LSVC does occur and can present as a mediastinal mass. CT angiographic or MRI scans clearly delineate these lesions.[23] An innominate vein aneurysm is rare (**Fig. 4**), with only about 14 cases reported in the literature.[24] It gives the appearance of the double aortic knob on the left side of the mediastinum and can be mistaken for a pseudocoarctation.[5] Hosein[24] reported respiratory distress in a 13-year-old postoperative patient

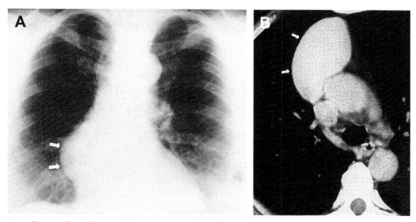

Fig. 3. (*A*) Chest radiograph with superior vena cava (SVC) aneurysm presenting as right hilar mass (*arrow*). (*B*) Contrast-enhanced chest CT scan of the same patient showing SVC aneurysm (*arrow*). (*From* Gozdziuk K, Czekajska-Chehab E, Wrona A, et al. Saccular aneurysm of the superior vena cava detected by CT and successfully treated with surgery. Ann Thorac Surg 2004;78(6):e94; with permission.)

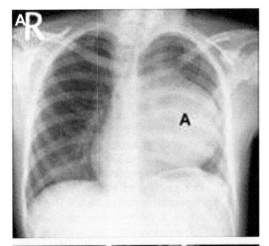

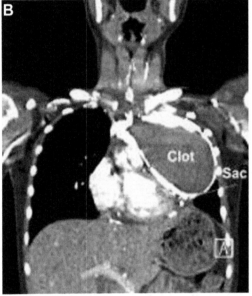

Fig. 4. Large innominate vein aneurysm on (*A*) chest radiograph and (*B*) CT scan. (*From* Hosein RB, Butler K, Miller P, et al. Innominate venous aneurysm presenting as a rapidly expanding mediastinal mass. Ann Thorac Surg 2007;84:641; with permission.)

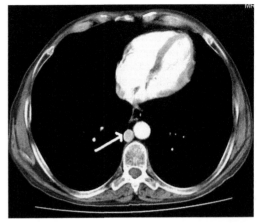

Fig. 5. Contrast-enhanced CT scan showing enlarged azygous vein (*arrow*). (*From* Martín-Malagón A, Bravo A, Arteaga I, et al. Ivor Lewis esophagectomy in a patient with enlarged azygos vein: a lesson to learn. Ann Thorac Surg 2008;85(1):327; with permission.)

caused by a rapidly enlarging innominate vein aneurysm that was treated successfully with surgical resection and reconstruction.

The azygous vein is considered enlarged when it is greater than 7 mm.[25] It gives the appearance of a right paratracheal mass or lymph node. A clue to differentiating this condition from other masses is the variability in size in the supine and erect positions. The vein is larger when the patient is in the supine position than when in the upright position.[4] Several clinical conditions that increase flow-through or venous pressure can lead to azygous vein enlargement (**Fig. 5**).[26] The most common causes include caval obstruction, hepatic vein obstruction, portal hypertension, inferior vena caval interruption with azygous continuation, pregnancy, and cardiac disease, including congestive heart failure, tricuspid disease, pericardial constriction, and tamponade.[5,27] Idiopathic aneurysmal enlargement occurs rarely.[28,29] Azygous vein varices (**Fig. 6**) or diverticula and aneurysms as large as 11 cm have been reported. Thrombosed large saccular aneurysms have been implicated as the cause of severe pulmonary hypertension because of chronic thromboembolism.[30]

Hemiazygous or azygous continuation can occur in patients who have situs solitus, but it commonly is associated with polysplenia or situs ambiguous syndromes. The hemiazygous vein also can enlarge in conditions that cause enlargement of the azygous vein. It appears as widening of the left paraspinous or paratracheal shadow.

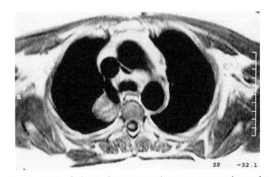

Fig. 6. MRI of chest demonstrating azygous vein varix of posterior mediastinum. (*From* Podbielski FJ, Sam II, AD, Halldorsson AO, et al. Giant azygos vein varix. Ann Thorac Surg 1997;63(4):1168; with permission.)

The supreme intercostal vein, which connects the left brachiocephalic vein and the hemiazygous vein, runs parallel to the aortic arch. Conditions that lead to increased flow or pressure in the thoracic venous system cause dilation of this vein. When it is enlarged, the radiographic appearance of this vein is referred to as the aortic nipple (**Fig. 7**).[5]

PULMONARY ARTERIAL SYSTEM

Pulmonary artery (PA) enlargement is frequently the result of a congenital heart anomaly or secondary to isolated pulmonary hypertension. Enlargement involves the pulmonary trunk and the main PAs. It presents radiographically as a middle mediastinal or perihilar mass. Conditions causing PA enlargement include pulmonary valve stenosis with or without tetralogy of Fallot (TOF), absent pulmonary valve (with or without TOF), Eisenmenger's syndrome, patent ductus arteriosus, PA shunt, and intracardiac shunt with large left-to-right component. Acute or chronic pulmonary embolism or idiopathic endocarditis[31] can cause PA enlargement. Postsurgical changes after systemic-to-PA shunts or transannular patches for repair of TOF can present as middle mediastinal or paratracheal masses.

In congenital PA stenosis, turbulence beyond the stenosis causes poststenotic dilatation in a fashion similar to that of poststenotic dilation with aortic stenosis. The direction of the jet is directed preferentially into the left PA and can lead to disproportionate enlargement of the left PA.[4]

Congenital absence of the pulmonary valve can occur as an isolated entity or in association with TOF (**Fig. 8**).[32] Affected infants present with

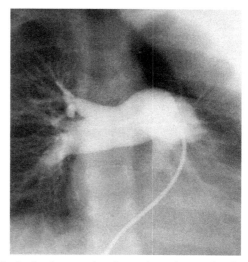

Fig. 8. Angiogram showing enlarged central pulmonary artery in absent pulmonary valve syndrome. (*From* Godart F, Houyel L, Lacour-Gayet F, et al. Absent pulmonary valve syndrome: surgical treatment and considerations. Ann Thorac Surg 1996;62(1):127; with permission.)

massive enlargement of the pulmonary trunk and main pulmonary arteries caused by the regurgitation across the annulus.[33,34] Children with this condition have the early signs and symptoms of right ventricular failure or cyanosis. The enlarged artery also can cause tracheobronchial compression. A reduction pulmonary arterioplasty with or without implantation of a valved conduit often is required to address the clinical problem.[35,36]

Idiopathic aneurysms of the PA are rare and can present with chest pain, shortness of breath, hemoptysis, or dissection (**Figs. 9** and **10**).[37–39] PA aneurysms also have been associated with collagen vascular disorders and systemic inflammatory states such as lupus. PA aneurysms are subject to the same complications as aortic aneurysms, and surgical intervention is recommended when they are large or symptomatic.[37] Dissections of the PA have been documented and successfully treated with surgical resection, although they represent the minority of cases.[39,40,41] Most reported cases were diagnosed postmortem.

Traumatic pulmonary pseudoaneurysms presenting as middle mediastinal masses also have been described and were managed successfully with coil embolization.[42] Unilateral pulmonary artery enlargement may be caused by a large pulmonary embolus. Referring to the medical history will help elucidate this as the cause of the mediastinal mass.

A PA sling occurs when the left PA originates directly from the posterior aspect of the right PA. PA sling commonly is associated with tracheal

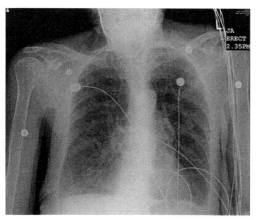

Fig. 7. Chest radiograph showing aortic nipple along aortic arch. (*Courtesy of* J. Domesek, MD, Philadelphia, PA.)

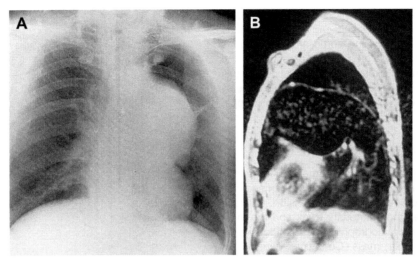

Fig. 9. (A) Chest radiograph of pulmonary artery aneurysm presenting as large mediastinal mass. (B) MRI showing large pulmonary artery aneurysm. (*From* Chen YF, Chiu CC, Lee CS. Giant aneurysm of main pulmonary artery. Ann Thorac Surg 1996;62(1):273; with permission.

stenosis. The left PA travels over the right main stem bronchus and then between the trachea to reach the left pulmonary hilum, forming a sling over the distal trachea and the right main stem and compressing these structures.[43,44] On a lateral plain film, a rounded density is seen between the trachea and esophagus. Infants present with stridor; results from a barium esophagram will confirm the diagnosis. Rarely, this anomaly is asymptomatic and presents as a right paratracheal mass in the older child or adult.[4] Surgical correction is either by translocation or reimplantation of the left PA with concomitant repair of any tracheal stenosis.

An aneurysm of the ductus arteriosus presents characteristically as a rounded mass adjacent to

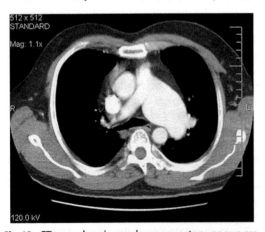

Fig. 10. CT scan showing pulmonary artery aneurysm. (*From* Foster JL, Bradley SM, Ikonomidis JS. Pulmonary artery aneurysm and coronary artery disease in the clinical presentation of Watson syndrome. Ann Thorac Surg 2006;82(2):741; with permission.)

the aortic knob and projects into the left mediastinum when viewed on plain film.[45] Infants who have this condition can present with respiratory distress at birth. Although it is a relatively rare condition, it can be associated with rupture, thromboembolism, and dissection. These aneurysms can present beyond the perinatal period and have been documented in patients as old as 73 years.[46] Local compressive forces can lead to tracheobronchial compression or hoarseness caused by compression of the recurrent laryngeal nerve. In older patients, calcifications can be present on plain film. Cases of nonpatent ductus arteriosus aneurysms have been documented.[45,46] Most authors recommend surgical intervention because of the risk of rupture, dissection, endocarditis, and pulmonary hypertension.

True aneurysms and pseudoaneurysms can present later after surgical correction of congenital heart disease. This situation has been documented in TOF patients who have received transannular patches, especially when pericardium is used.[47] The true aneurysm or pseudoaneurysm presents as an enlargement of the right ventricular border on chest radiographs in lateral views. Systemic-to-pulmonary artery shunts for cyanotic heart disease can cause aneurysmal dilation of the PA, particularly if the flow through the shunt is excessive.[5] The Potts shunt is particularly prone to this complication, causing left pulmonary aneurysms.

PULMONARY VENOUS SYSTEM

Anomalies of the pulmonary venous system that can present as mediastinal masses include partial

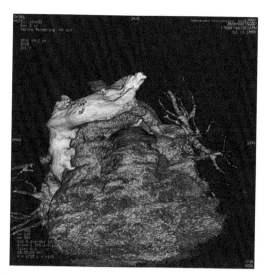

Fig. 11. CT scan showing partial anomalous pulmonary venous return of the superior pulmonary vein. (*Courtesy of* J. Domesek, MD, Philadelphia, PA.)

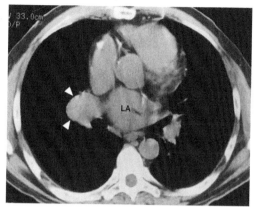

Fig. 12. CT scan showing right superior pulmonary vein aneurysm (*arrow*). (*From* Sirivella S, Gielchinsky I. Pulmonary venous aneurysm presenting as a mediastinal mass in ischemic cardiomyopathy. Ann Thorac Surg 1999;68(1):242; with permission.)

and total anomalous venous return (**Fig. 11**), pulmonary venous varix, and pulmonary venous confluence. Partial anomalous venous return more commonly involves the right lung in association with an atrial septal defect. Rarely, the left upper lobe vein connects to the left innominate vein and presents radiologically as a density lateral to the aortic arch. This finding has to be differentiated from a persistent LSVC.[5]

In type 1 or supercardiac total anomalous pulmonary venous connection, the classic chest radiograph finding is described as a "figure eight" or snowman appearance caused by dilation of the venous structures involved.[4] Often, a vertical vein connects the venous confluence to the innominate vein or LSVC. Partial or total obstruction will cause severe symptoms in infants, creating a surgical emergency. Cases of adults presenting with only severe pulmonary stenosis and suggestion of mediastinal mass have been reported.[48]

A pulmonary venous varix is a local dilation of one or more pulmonary veins with normal drainage to the left atrium. It can be congenital or acquired. Congenital varices are generally asymptomatic and do not change in size over the years unless associated with pulmonary hypertension. Acquired forms present with symptoms of the associated disease, are usually seen in mitral valve disease,[49] and can regress after mitral valve replacement. Pulmonary varix will present as a perihilar or middle mediastinal mass on a chest radiograph. Pulmonary vein aneurysm is rare (**Fig. 12**).[50] Sirivella and colleagues[51] reported one involving the right superior pulmonary vein in a patient who

had ischemic cardiomyopathy that presented as a middle mediastinal mass.

A pulmonary venous confluence is produced when the upper, lower, or middle lobe veins come together before entering the left atrium.[4] This formation simulates a middle mediastinal mass.

SYSTEMIC ARTERIAL SYSTEM

Vascular lesions of the arterial system that present as mediastinal masses span the spectrum from

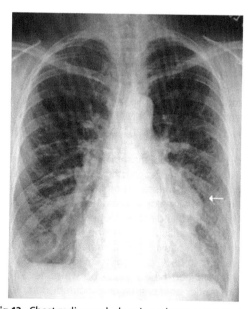

Fig. 13. Chest radiograph showing a large coronary aneurysm presenting as a left para-cardiac mass. (*From* Agarwal R, Jeevanandam V, Jolly N. Surgical treatment of a giant coronary artery aneurysm: a modified approach. Ann Thorac Surg 2007;84(4):1392; with permission.)

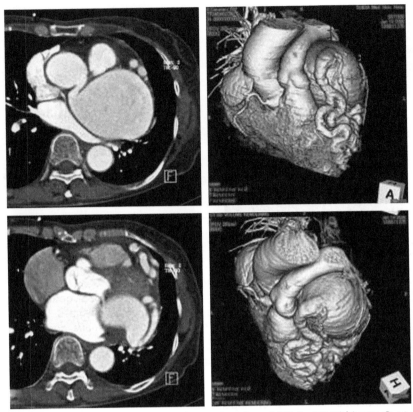

Fig. 14. Large left main coronary artery aneurysm. (*From* Matsubayashi K, Asai T, Nishimura O, et al. Giant coronary artery aneurysm in the left main coronary artery: a novel surgical procedure. Ann Thorac Surg 2008;85(6):2131; with permission.)

congenital lesions to acquired and traumatic lesions of the thoracic aorta. In the adult patient, the most common vascular lesions are aneurysms of the thoracic aorta. The differentiation of aneurysms of the thoracic aorta from other mediastinal masses is readily apparent on diagnostic images. Causes of aortic aneurysms are atherosclerosis, trauma, and inflammatory or cystic medial necrosis. Acute aortic dissection can present with nonspecific radiographic findings that simulate a mediastinal mass. Prompt recognition of the lesion can make a dramatic difference in the natural history of this disease. Depending on the location of the dissection in the thorax and the constellation of symptoms, immediate surgical intervention (type A) or medical management alone (uncomplicated type B) may be warranted. Thoracic aortic aneurysms are located commonly below the level of the ligamentum arteriosus, then the arch, followed by the ascending aorta.

Although other portions of the aorta also can be involved, post-traumatic chronic pseudoaneurysms typically occur at the aortic isthmus and may present as a mediastinal mass. This condition results from undiagnosed acute aortic injury caused by trauma where acceleration/deceleration forces are applied to the aorta.

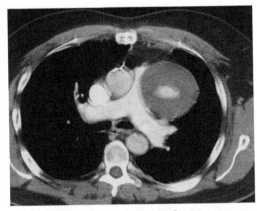

Fig. 15. Large saphenous vein graft aneurysm compressing main pulmonary artery. (*From* Mitchell MB, Campbell DN. Pulmonary artery compression by a giant aorto–coronary vein graft aneurysm. Ann Thorac Surg 2000;69(3):948; with permission.)

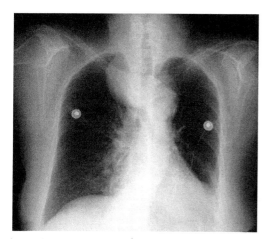

Fig. 16. Large aneurysm of Kommerell's diverticulum. (*From* Kouchoukos NT, Masetti P. Aberrant subclavian artery and Kommerell aneurysm: surgical treatment with a standard approach. J Thorac Cardiovasc Surg 2007;133(4):889; with permission.)

The diagnosis and management of thoracic aortic aneurysms and dissections have been reviewed by several authors.[52–54]

Other less common vascular arterial lesions include coronary aneurysms or fistulas; poststenotic dilation of the ascending aorta in adult and congenital aorta stenosis; tortuosity or aneurysms of the innominate artery, right aortic arch, and cervical aortic arch; and coarctation of the aorta.

Tortuosity or buckling of the innominate artery can present as a superior mediastinal or apical lung mass.[55] Tortuosity is common in older individuals and can be seen in up to 20% of patients who have hypertension, atherosclerosis, or both. The superior mediastinal density seen on imaging represents the artery itself or a displaced SVC in the cervical region.[4]

Coronary artery aneurysms have been reported to occur in about 0.4% to 5% of patients undergoing coronary angiography.[56] They are usually atherosclerotic in nature, but syphilitic, mycotic, or Kawasaki disease-related cases all have been documented and often involve the right coronary artery. A coronary artery aneurysm presents as a left or right paracardiac mass, depending on the artery involved (**Figs. 13** and **14**).[57,58] It can be asymptomatic, but can rupture, causing myocardial ischemia, and it can be complicated by endocarditis. As such, surgical resection is recommended.[59]

A coronary artery fistula is a congenital malformation in which the coronary artery drains into one of the cardiac chambers, the coronary sinus, the vena cavae, or the PA. More than 90% drain into the right heart, creating a left-to-right shunt. The remainder drain into the left heart. The involved artery, often the right, can become tortuous and aneurysmal over time. The fistula, like an aneurysm, is prone to rupture (rare), infection, and myocardial ischemia.[60,61]

A saphenous vein graft aneurysm is rare. It can be a true or false aneurysm and may present as a paracardiac mass (**Fig. 15**).[62] It can present as

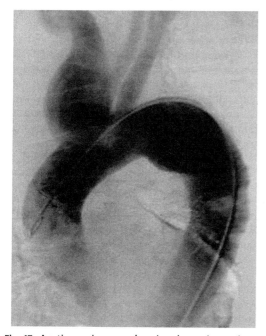

Fig. 17. Aortic angiogram showing large innominate artery aneurysm. (*From* McFarland JJ, Kahn MB, Bellows CF, et al. Superior vena cava syndrome caused by aneurysm of the innominate artery. Ann Thorac Surg 1995;59(1):228; with permission.)

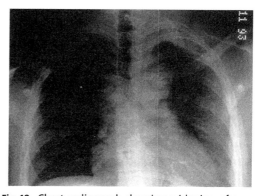

Fig. 18. Chest radiograph showing widening of superior mediastinum due to innominate artery aneurysm. (*From* Halpin DP, Nicholson J, Blakemore WS, Harlan JL. Innominate artery pseudoaneurysm presenting as a widened mediastinum. J Thorac Cardiovasc Surg 1995;109(2):390; with permission.)

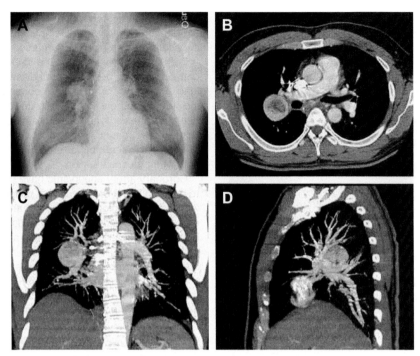

Fig. 19. (*A*) Chest radiograph showing right hilar mass. (*B–D*) Contrast-enhanced CT scan depicting this mass as a bronchial aneurysm. (*From* Lin J, Wood DE. Bronchial artery aneurysm refractory to transcatheter embolization. Ann Thorac Surg 2008;86(1):307; with permission.)

early as 10 days after coronary artery bypass surgery[63] and can be large.[64] Surgical intervention is required to prevent rupture, myocardial infarction, embolization, or death.

An aneurysm of the sinus of Valsalva usually involves the noncoronary and right coronary sinuses. It also appears as a paracardiac mass when massively enlarged. The aneurysm can cause conduction abnormalities, angina, aortic or mitral incompetence, and right ventricular outflow obstruction from the effect of the mass. Alternatively, it can rupture, usually into the right cardiac chambers.[65] Surgical resection is warranted when symptoms are present.

A left ventricular aneurysm can be congenital or acquired and appears as a paracardiac mass on plain chest radiograph. Congenital aneurysms can occur as part of the pentalogy of Cantrell's syndrome, whereas acquired aneurysms are usually a result of a myocardial infarction.[66,67]

ARCH ANOMALIES

Anomalies of the congenital aortic arch involve the abnormal location of the arch or branching abnormalities. Any of these can present as a mediastinal mass. They include a right aortic arch, vascular rings, cervical aortic arch, and coarctation.

A right aortic arch is reported to occur in 0.5% of patients and often is mistaken for a right paratracheal mass. The aortic arch projects into the right superior mediastinum. Most patients with a right aortic arch have a left innominate artery and are asymptomatic. A few patients have an aberrant left subclavian artery, which can cause dysphagia because of its retroesophageal course. The trachea is deviated to the left, and the SVC to the right.[4] Kommerell's diverticulum often is associated with an aberrant left subclavian artery (**Fig. 16**). The diverticulum can be become quite enlarged and cause local compression (dysphagia) or rupture.[68] Surgical intervention is recommended for large or symptomatic aneurysms.[69]

A left aortic arch with an aberrant right subclavian artery also can present as a right paratracheal mass. The course of the subclavian artery is usually posterior to the esophagus, but it also can travel between the esophagus and trachea or in front of the trachea. The radiographic appearance is more common in older individuals.[5] Kommerell's diverticulum also can be found with this arch anomaly. Although this condition is often asymptomatic in children, in adults, aneurysms of the aberrant subclavian, the diverticulum, or a prominent diverticulum alone can cause dysphagia.[5] Posterior indentation of the esophagus, seen on a barium esophagram, is seen in the lateral projection.

The four main types of vascular rings are double aortic arch with mirror image branching, right aortic artery with left ligamentum, innominate artery compression, and a PA sling.

A double aortic arch with mirror image branching can present as a mediastinal mass. If both arches are of equal size, then the right arch typically is read as a right paratracheal mass. The right arch is, however, often larger than the left. Infants present with stridor, and surgical division of the smaller arch is indicated to relieve the compression.[70]

When the innominate artery originates further leftward than usual, it can cause compression of the trachea and is seen radiographically as an anterior mediastinal mass indenting the trachea. It is classified as a partial vascular ring. Bronchoscopy is required to confirm the diagnosis.[43]

Innominate artery aneurysms are rare and can involve the proximal or entire innominate artery (**Fig. 17**). True and false aneurysms have been reported.[71–73] The chest radiograph will show widening of the superior mediastinum (**Fig. 18**).[74] Degenerative, mycotic, traumatic, connective tissue disorders, or extension of arch pathologic conditions have been implicated in innominate artery aneurysms. McFarland and colleagues[75] reported sudden rupture of an innominate artery aneurysm leading to acute SVC syndrome in one patient. Bower and colleagues[72] recommend operative treatment for all symptomatic and asymptomatic aneurysms because of the increased risk of rupture, thrombosis, and peripheral embolization. Aneurysm of the innominate artery may present on clinical examination as a pulsatile mass at the base of the neck or cause pain, hoarseness, Horner's syndrome, or dysphagia.

Rarely, the aortic arch can extend into the cervical region and appears as a superior mediastinal mass. This condition is referred to as a cervical aortic arch and is generally an asymptomatic finding. Some patients present with dysphagia or stridor even when the arch is not enlarged. The cervical arch can become aneurysmal and is subject to rupture like aneurysms elsewhere.[43]

Aortic coarctation is a congenital lesion that often is diagnosed and corrected in infancy. About 20% of patients are diagnosed in adolescence or as adults. Long-standing coarctation can present as a mediastinal mass when the left subclavian artery becomes dilated, and the aorta distal to the area of constriction also dilates. This configuration has been called the "figure 3" sign when seen on a radiograph.[55] If the coarctation goes uncorrected, the descending thoracic aorta beyond the area of constriction also can become aneurysmal, with an incidence as high as 20% by the third decade.[76] The aorta can kink or buckle in the area of the ligamentum arteriosum if it becomes elongated. This condition gives the impression of coarctation and hence is referred to as pseudo-coarctation, because no pressure gradient occurs across the area of kinking.[55] The aorta can dilate proximally and distally to the area of kinking. The dilated proximally aorta projects into the superior mediastinum and appears as a left superior mediastinal mass.

A bronchial artery aneurysm is a rare lesion that can present as a middle mediastinal mass (**Fig. 19**).[77] The finding can be an incidental finding, or it can present with rupture and shock.[78]

The clinical presentation and radiographic appearance can mimic aortic dissection or a ruptured aortic aneurysm.[79] A life-threatening hemorrhage from a ruptured bronchial aneurysm can occur; prompt recognition and management can be life saving.[80]

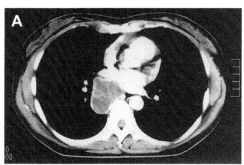
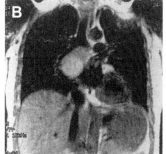

Fig. 20. (*A*) CT scan of chest with hemangioma of posterior mediastinum. (*B*) MRI of chest with same lesion. (*From* Sakamoto K, Okita M, Kumagiri H, et al. Sclerosing hemangioma isolated to the mediastinum. Ann Thorac Surg 2003;75(3):1022; with permission.)

Incidentally detected mediastinal bronchial artery aneurysms should be considered unstable regardless of size.[78,79] Open repair and catheter embolization are options for management.

VASCULAR TUMORS

Hemangiomas have been described in the mediastinum (**Fig. 20**).[81] They can occur as an isolated lesion or within an intracardiac location. They have been described in association with the SVC[82] and the coronary artery.[83] Hemangiomas often are mixed tumors and are associated with lymphagiomas.[84] In this case, they are referred to as lymphangioma–hemangioma. Besides causing local mass effect, they can present with spontaneous hemorrhage or with the Kasabach-Merritt syndrome.[85] MRI is the preferred imaging modality and will delineate the vascular nature of the mass if the diagnosis is in question. Surgical resection and nonoperative therapy with pulse steroids and interferon are options for managing mediastinal hemangiomas.[83,86] Other vascular neoplasms that must be considered when evaluating a vascular mass are angiosarcoma and hemangiopericytoma.

SUMMARY

Most mediastinal masses seen on thoracic imaging are of solid tumor origin. As such, vascular lesions of the mediastinum can be mistaken for, or misinterpreted as, one of these more common mediastinal masses. This article stresses the importance of considering vascular entities in the differential diagnosis of mediastinal masses.

REFERENCES

1. Gozdziuk K, Czekajska-Chehab E, Wrona A, et al. Saccular aneurysm of the superior vena cava detected by computed tomography and successfully treated with surgery. Ann Thorac Surg 2004;78(6): e94–5.
2. Lyons HA, Calvy GL, Sammons BP. The diagnosis and classification of mediastinal masses. 1. A study of 782 cases. Ann Intern Med 1959;51:897–932.
3. Shields TW, LoCicero J III, Ponn RB, et al. The mediastinum, its compartments, and the mediastinal lymph nodes. In: Shields TW, Ponn JB, Rusch VW, editors. 6th edition, General thoracic surgery, vol. 2. Philadelphia: Lippincott Williams & Wilkins; 2005. p. 2343–6.
4. Kelley MJ, Mannes EJ, Ravin CE. Mediastinal masses of vascular origin. A review. J Thorac Cardiovasc Surg 1978;76(4):559–72.
5. Shields TW, LoCicero J III, Ponn RB, et al. Vascular masses of the mediastinum. In: Shields TW, Ponn JB, Rusch VW, editors. 6th edition, General thoracic surgery, vol. 2. Philadelphia: Lippincott Williams & Wilkins; 2005. p. 2523–44.
6. Bossert T, Gummert JF, Mohr FW. Giant cystic lymphangioma of the mediastinum. Eur J Cardiothorac Surg 2002;21(2):340.
7. Adil A, Ksiyer M. Unusual mediastinal cystic lymphangioma. Apropos of a case and review of the literature. Ann Radiol (Paris) 1996;39(6):249–52.
8. Okubo T, Okayasu T, Osaka Y, et al. Surgical analysis of mediastinal lymphangioma—analysis of 7 cases. Nippon Kyobu Geka Gakkai Zasshi 1992; 40(4):583–6.
9. Bilgin M, Akçali Y, Oğuzkaya F, et al. Mediastinal cystic lymphangioma: a rare mediastinal tumor. Turkish respiratory Journal 2004;5(3):187–8.
10. Teramoto K, Suzumura Y. Mediastinal cavernous lymphangioma in an adult. Gen Thorac Cardiovasc Surg 2008;56(2):88–90.
11. Jougon J, Laborde MN, Parrens M, et al. Cystic lymphangioma of the heart mimicking a mediastinal tumor. Eur J Cardiothorac Surg 2002;22(3):476–8.
12. Okazaki T, Iwatani S, Yanai T, et al. Treatment of lymphangioma in children: our experience of 128 cases. J Pediatr Surg 2007;42(2):386–9.
13. Daya SK, Gowda RM, Gowda MR, et al. Thoracic cystic lymphangioma (cystic hygroma): a chest pain syndrome—a case report. Angiology 2004; 55(5):561–4.
14. Oshikiri T, Morikawa T, Jinushi E, et al. Five cases of the lymphangioma of the mediastinum in adult. Ann Thorac Cardiovasc Surg 2001;7(2):103–5.
15. Degenhardt P, Dieckow B, Mau H. Huge intra- and extrathoracic lymphangioma in a baby successfully treated by sclerotherapy with OK-432. Eur J Pediatr Surg 2006;16(3):197–200.
16. Wong PS, Goldstraw P. Left superior vena cava: a pitfall in computed tomographic diagnosis with surgical implications. Ann Thorac Surg 1990;50(4):656–7.
17. Varma PK, Dharan BS, Ramachandran P, et al. Superior vena caval aneurysm. Interact Cardiovasc Thorac Surg 2003;2(3):331–3.
18. Joseph AE, Donaldson JS, Reynolds M. Neck and thorax venous aneurysm: association with cystic hygroma. Radiology 1989;170(1 Pt 1):109–12.
19. Kouchoukos NT, Blackstone EH, Doty DB, et al. Atrial septal defect and partial anomalous venous connection. In: Kirklin/Barratt-Boyes cardiac surgery. 3rd edition. Philadelphia: Churchill Livingstone; 2003. p. 715–51.
20. Gandhi SK, Siewers R. Anomalies of systemic venous drainage. In: Kaiser LR, Kron IL, Spray TL, editors. Mastery of cardiothoracic surgery. Philadelphia: Lippincott Williams & Wilkins; 2007. p. 708–15.
21. Kouchoukos NT, Blackstone EH, Doty DB, et al. Cor triatriatum. In: Kirklin/Barratt-Boyes cardiac surgery. 3rd edition. Philadelphia: Churchill Livingstone; 2003. p. 781–9.

22. Pahwa R, Kumar A. Persistent left superior vena cava: an intensivist's experience and review of the literature. South Med J 2003;96(5):528–9.

23. Teske DW, Davis JT, Allen HD. Cavopulmonary anastomotic aneurysm: a complication in pulsatile pulmonary arteries. Ann Thorac Surg 1994;57(6):1661–3 [discussion: 1663–4].

24. Hosein RB, Butler K, Miller P, et al. Innominate venous aneurysm presenting as a rapidly expanding mediastinal mass. Ann Thorac Surg 2007;84(2): 640–2.

25. Heitzman ER. Radiologic appearance of the azygos vein in cardiovascular disease. Circulation 1973; 47(3):628–34.

26. Martín-Malagón A, Bravo A, Arteaga I, et al. Ivor Lewis esophagectomy in a patient with enlarged azygos vein: a lesson to learn. Ann Thorac Surg 2008;85(1):326–8.

27. Podbielski FJ, Sam AD II, Halldorsson AO, et al. Giant azygos vein varix. Ann Thorac Surg 1997; 63(4):1167–9.

28. Watanabe A, Kusajima K, Aisaka N, et al. Idiopathic saccular azygos vein aneurysm. Ann Thorac Surg 1998;65(5):1459–61.

29. Lena H, Desrues B, Heresbach D, et al. Azygos vein aneurysm: contribution of transesophageal echography. Ann Thorac Surg 1996;61(4):1253–5.

30. Nakamura Y, Nakano K, Nakatani H, et al. Surgical exclusion of a thrombosed azygos vein aneurysm causing pulmonary embolism. J Thorac Cardiovasc Surg 2007;133(3):834–5.

31. Bozkurt AK, Oztunc F, Akman C, et al. Multiple pulmonary artery aneurysms due to infective endocarditis. Ann Thorac Surg 2003;75(2):593–6.

32. Godart F, Houyel L, Lacour-Gayet F, et al. Absent pulmonary valve syndrome: surgical treatment and considerations. Ann Thorac Surg 1996;62(1): 136–42.

33. Duncan BW, Mee RBB. Tetralogy of Fallot with pulmonary stenosis. In: Sellke FW, del Nido PJ, Swanson SJ, editors. 7th edition, Sabiston and Spencer surgery of the chest, vol. 2. Philadelphia: Elsevier/WB Saunders; 2005. p. 2013–34.

34. Kouchoukos NT, Blackstone EH, Doty DB, et al. Ventricular septal defect with pulmonary stenosis or atresia. In: Kirklin/Barratt-Boyes cardiac surgery. 3rd edition. Philadelphia: Churchill Livingstone; 2003. p. 946–1073.

35. Jaquiss RDB. Tetralogy of Fallot. In: Kaiser LR, Kron IL, Spray TL, editors. Mastery of cardiothoracic surgery. Philadelphia: Lippincott Williams & Wilkins; 2007. p. 907–15.

36. Karl TR, Musumeci F, de Leval M, et al. Surgical treatment of absent pulmonary valve syndrome. J Thorac Cardiovasc Surg 1986;91(4):590–7.

37. Rajpurohit V, Patil PK. Idiopathic pulmonary artery aneurysm. Bombay Hosp J. Available at: http:// www.bhj.org/journal/2005_4701_jan/html/case_ Idiopathic.htm. Accessed August 21, 2008.

38. Aroussi AA, Redai M, El Ouardi F, et al. Bilateral pulmonary artery aneurysm in Behçet syndrome: report of two operative cases. J Thorac Cardiovasc Surg 2005;129(5):1170–1.

39. Senbaklavaci O, Kaneko Y, Bartunek A, et al. Rupture and dissection in pulmonary artery aneurysms: incidence, cause, and treatment—review and case report. J Thorac Cardiovasc Surg 2001; 121(5):1006–8.

40. Deb SJ, Zehr KJ, Shields RC. Idiopathic pulmonary artery aneurysm. Ann Thorac Surg 2005;80(4): 1500–2.

41. Wuyts WA, Herijgers P, Budts W, et al. Extensive dissection of the pulmonary artery treated with combined heart–lung transplantation. J Thorac Cardiovasc Surg 2006;132(1):205–6.

42. Block M, Lefkowitz T, Ravenel J, et al. Endovascular coil embolization for acute management of traumatic pulmonary artery pseudoaneurysm. J Thorac Cardiovasc Surg 2004;128(5):784–5.

43. Austin EH III, Kavarana MN. Vascular rings, slings, and other arch anomalies. In: Kaiser LR, Kron IL, Spray TL, editors. Mastery of cardiothoracic surgery. 2nd edition. Philadelphia: Lippincott Williams & Wilkins; 2007. p. 722–38.

44. Backer CL, Idriss FS, Holinger LD, et al. Pulmonary artery sling. Results of surgical repair in infancy. J Thorac Cardiovasc Surg 1992;103(4): 683–91.

45. Cheng TO. Aneurysm of a nonpatent ductus arteriosus. An unusual cause of mediastinal mass. Dis Chest 1969;55(6):497–500.

46. Myojin K, Ishibashi Y, Ishii K, et al. Aneurysm of the nonpatent ductus arteriosus in the adult—a report of the case and review of the literature. Jpn J Thorac Cardiovasc Surg 1998;46(9):882–8.

47. Seybold-Epting W, Chiariello L, Hallman GL, et al. Aneurysm of pericardial right ventricular outflow tract patches. Ann Thorac Surg 1977;24(3):237–40.

48. Pastore JO, Akins CW, Zir LM, et al. Total anomalous pulmonary venous connection and severe pulmonic stenosis in a 52-year-old man. Circulation 1977; 55(1):206–9.

49. Shida T, Ohashi H, Nakamura K, et al. Pulmonary varices associated with mitral valve disease: a case report and survey of the literature. Ann Thorac Surg 1982;34(4):452–6.

50. DeBoer DA, Margolis ML, Livornese D, et al. Pulmonary venous aneurysm presenting as a middle mediastinal mass. Ann Thorac Surg 1996;61(4): 1261–2.

51. Sirivella S, Gielchinsky I. Pulmonary venous aneurysm presenting as a mediastinal mass in ischemic cardiomyopathy. Ann Thorac Surg 1999;68(1): 241–3.

52. Crawford ES, Svensson LG, Coselli JS, et al. Surgical treatment of aneurysm and/or dissection of the ascending aorta, transverse aortic arch, and ascending aorta and transverse aortic arch. Factors influencing survival in 717 patients. J Thorac Cardiovasc Surg 1989;98:659–73.

53. Bavaria JE, Appoo JJ, Makaroun MS, et al. Endovascular stent grafting versus open surgical repair of descending thoracic aortic aneurysms in low-risk patients: a multicenter comparative trial. J Thorac Cardiovasc Surg 2007;133(2):369–77.

54. Dapunt OE, Galla JD, Sadeghi AM, et al. The natural history of thoracic aortic aneurysms. J Thorac Cardiovasc Surg 1994;107(5):1323–32 [discussion: 1332–3].

55. Smyth PT, Edwards JE. Pseudocoarctation, kinking, or buckling of the aorta. Circulation 1972;46(5):1027–32.

56. Syed M, Lesch M. Coronary artery aneurysm: a review. Prog Cardiovasc Dis 1997;40(1):77–84.

57. Agarwal R, Jeevanandam V, Jolly N. Surgical treatment of a giant coronary artery aneurysm: a modified approach. Ann Thorac Surg 2007;84(4):1392–4.

58. Matsubayashi K, Asai T, Nishimura O, et al. Giant coronary artery aneurysm in the left main coronary artery: a novel surgical procedure. Ann Thorac Surg 2008;85(6):2130–2.

59. Baek WK, Kim JT, Yoon YH, et al. Huge sinus of valsalva aneurysm causing mitral valve incompetence. Ann Thorac Surg 2002;73(6):1975–7.

60. Kouchoukos NT, Blackstone EH, Doty DB, et al. Congenital anomalies of the coronary artery. In: Kirklin/Barratt-Boyes cardiac surgery. 3rd edition. Philadelphia: Churchill Livingstone; 2003. p. 1240–63.

61. Gaynor JW. Coronary anomalies in children. In: Kaiser LR, Kron IL, Spray TL, editors. Mastery of cardiothoracic surgery. 2nd edition. Philadelphia: Lippincott Williams & Wilkins; 2007. p. 959–72.

62. Mitchell MB, Campbell DN. Pulmonary artery compression by a giant aortocoronary vein graft aneurysm. Ann Thorac Surg 2000;69(3):948–9.

63. Trop I, Samson L, Cordeau MP, et al. Anterior mediastinal mass in a patient with prior saphenous vein coronary artery bypass grafting. Chest 1999;115(2):572–6.

64. Kalimi R, Palazzo RS, Graver LM. Giant aneurysm of saphenous vein graft to coronary artery compressing the right atrium. Ann Thorac Surg 1999;68(4):1433–7.

65. Luckraz H, Naik M, Jenkins G, et al. Repair of a sinus of valsalva aneurysm that had ruptured into the pulmonary artery. J Thorac Cardiovasc Surg 2004;127(6):1823–5.

66. Fauza DO, Allmendinger N, Wilson JM. Congenital diaphragmatic hernia. In: Sellke FW, del Nido PJ, Swanson SJ, editors. 7th edition, Sabiston and Spencer surgery of the chest, vol. 1. Philadelphia: Elsevier/WB Saunders; 2005. p. 517–45.

67. Kouchoukos NT, Blackstone EH, Doty DB, et al. Left ventricular aneurysm. In: Kirklin/Barratt-Boyes cardiac surgery. 3rd edition. Philadelphia: Churchill Livingstone; 2003. p. 437–55.

68. Kouchoukos NT, Masetti P. Aberrant subclavian artery and Kommerell aneurysm: surgical treatment with a standard approach. J Thorac Cardiovasc Surg 2007;133(4):888–92.

69. Cina CS, Althani H, Pasenau J, et al. Kommerell's diverticulum and right-sided aortic arch: a cohort study and review of the literature. J Vasc Surg 2004;39(1):131–9.

70. Burke RP. Patent ductus arteriosus and vascular rings. In: Sellke FW, del Nido PJ, Swanson SJ, editors. 7th edition, Sabiston and Spencer surgery of the chest, vol. 1. Philadelphia: Elsevier/WB Saunders; 2005. p. 1897–912.

71. Kieffer E, Chiche L, Koskas F, et al. Aneurysms of the innominate artery: surgical treatment of 27 patients. J Vasc Surg 2001;34(2):222–8.

72. Bower TC, Pairolero PC, Hallett JW Jr, et al. Brachiocephalic aneurysm: the case for early recognition and repair. Ann Vasc Surg 1991;5(2):125–32.

73. Takach TJ, Lalka SG. Innominate artery aneurysm: axial reconstruction via a cervical approach. J Vasc Surg 2007;46(6):1267–9.

74. Halpin DP, Nicholson J, Blakemore WS, et al. Innominate artery pseudoaneurysm presenting as a widened mediastinum. J Thorac Cardiovasc Surg 1995;109(2):390–1.

75. McFarland JJ, Kahn MB, Bellows CF, et al. Superior vena cava syndrome caused by aneurysm of the innominate artery. Ann Thorac Surg 1995;59(1):227–9.

76. Kouchoukos NT, Blackstone EH, Doty DB, et al. Coarctation of the aorta and interrupted aortic arch. In: Kirklin/Barratt-Boyes cardiac surgery. 3rd edition. Philadelphia: Churchill Livingstone; 2003. p. 1315–400.

77. Lin J, Wood DE. Bronchial artery aneurysm refractory to transcatheter embolization. Ann Thorac Surg 2008;86(1):306–8.

78. Suen HC, Dumontier CC, Boeren J, et al. Ruptured bronchial artery aneurysm associated with sarcoidosis. J Thorac Cardiovasc Surg 2003;125(5):1153–4.

79. Kalangos A, Khatchatourian G, Panos A, et al. Ruptured mediastinal bronchial artery aneurysm: a dilemma of diagnosis and therapeutic approach. J Thorac Cardiovasc Surg 1997;114(5):853–6.

80. Sanchez E, Alados P, Zurera L, et al. Bronchial artery aneurysm treated with aortic stent graft and fibrin sealant. Ann Thorac Surg 2007;83(2):693–5.

81. Sakamoto K, Okita M, Kumagiri H, et al. Sclerosing hemangioma isolated to the mediastinum. Ann Thorac Surg 2003;75(3):1021–3.

82. Demmy TL, Krasna MJ, Detterbeck FC, et al. Multi-center VATS experience with mediastinal tumors. Ann Thorac Surg 1998;66(1):187–92.

83. Turkoz R, Gulcan O, Oguzkurt L, et al. Surgical treatment of a huge cavernous hemangioma surrounding the right coronary artery. Ann Thorac Surg 2005;79(5):1765–7.

84. Riquet M, Briere J, Le Pimpec-Barthes F, et al. Lym-phangiohemangioma of the mediastinum. Ann Thorac Surg 1997;64(5):1476–8.

85. Iwami D, Shimaoka S, Mochizuki I, et al. Kaposiform hemangioendpothelioma of the mediastinum in a 7-month-old boy: a case report. J Pediatr Surg 2006;41(8):1486–8.

86. Kumar P, Judson I, Nicholson AG, et al. Medias-tinal hemangioma: successful treatment by al-pha-2a interferon and postchemotherapy resection. J Thorac Cardiovasc Surg 2002; 124(2):404–6.

Combined Cervicothoracic Approaches for Complex Mediastinal Masses

Clemens Aigner, MD, Mir Ali Reza Hoda, MD,
Walter Klepetko, MD*

KEYWORDS

- Cervicothoracic approach • Mediastinal tumor
- Extended resection • Anterior approach
- Posterior approach

The cervicothoracic junction is an anatomic complex region that contains important neurovascular structures and the central routes of the airway and upper digestive tract. Masses arising in either compartment—the mediastinum or the cervical region—may involve the other one extensively, requiring a combined surgical approach to achieve complete resection. The choice of the most appropriate approach is therefore crucial and requires careful preoperative planning.

Appropriate exposure is crucial to obtain good surgical results, however at the same time difficult to achieve, because access is limited by the anatomic barrier of the rib cage and the clavicles, which protect the sensitive area. This in addition is paralleled by the need to preserve a maximum of important functional structures, to maintain their diligent functional interaction.

The histologic origin of masses encountered in this region derives from a large and heterogeneous variety of different entities. It comprises malignant tumors of primary and metastatic origin, and benign lesions with expansive local growth patterns.[1]

ANATOMIC CONSIDERATIONS

The central structures of the neck are the trachea, located in an anterior position in the midline axis, together with the esophagus posterior and the recurrent laryngeal nerves laterally. These are paralleled in close vicinity by the central neurovascular bundle including the carotid artery, the jugular vein, and the vagus nerve. The lateral part of the neck can be divided further in three compartments based on the insertion of the scalene muscles. In the anterior compartment in front of the anterior scalene muscle, the subclavian and internal jugular veins are located, together with the sternocleidomastoid and omohyoid muscles. In the middle compartment between anterior and middle scalene muscle, the subclavian artery, the trunks of the brachial plexus, and the phrenic nerve are found. In the posterior compartment between middle and posterior scalene muscles, the nerve roots of the brachial plexus are situated as well as the stellate ganglion and the vertebral column. The mediastinum itself can be divided in the four known compartments, the superior, anterior, middle, and posterior compartments.

Most combined cervicothoracic masses extend along the midline axis into the mediastinum either in the anterior or posterior routes. A somewhat smaller minority, however, bridges the infra- and supraclavicular spaces and sometimes extends on the thoracic side into the lungs. Among them, the most important entities are primary tumors of the lung, extending into the chest wall at the level of the first rib, the so-called

Medical University of Vienna, Waehinger Guertel 18-20, 1090 Vienna, Austria
* Corresponding author.
E-mail address: walter.klepetko@meduniwien.ac.at (W. Klepetko).

Thorac Surg Clin 19 (2009) 107–112
doi:10.1016/j.thorsurg.2008.09.011

Pancoast-Tobias tumors,[2] which will not be discussed in detail here.

Tumors or masses occurring in a cervicothoracic position can have a large variety in their histologic origin. Although there is a preference of tumors of certain histology to arise in one of the described compartments, most can arise in any other surrounding compartment also. By principle, one has to distinguish between benign and malignant lesions and primary and metastatic lesions. The spectrum of primary lesions found in these locations is large and includes neurogenic tumors, sarcomatous tumors, lymphomas, thymomas, and many others.[3] Accordingly, the indication for surgical resection varies, and especially in malignant lesions, surgery frequently is part of a multimodality treatment, which starts with induction chemotherapy or chemoradiotherapy.

Metastatic lesions can occur as single solid masses or present as multiple involved lymph nodes. Again, the indication for surgical resection varies enormously, according to the underlying entity, and therefore cannot be discussed in every detail. even extensive lymph node involvement, however, sometimes can be an indication for surgical resection, especially in case of germ cell tumors or well-differentiated thyroid malignancies.

Benign lesions in this area are comprised mainly of cysts of various origins or occasionally others like diverticula or aneurysms.

SURGICAL APPROACHES: GENERAL ASPECTS

Adequate access is important for any operation in a critical region such as the cervicothoracic junction. The anatomic location of the mass to be resected usually dictates either an anterior or posterior approach. The choice of the particular approach, however, has to be performed with respect to several other important aspects. The incision has to be wide enough to allow for complete control of the major vessels. The functional integrity of the sternoclavicular junction and the upper end of the rib cage should be preserved as well as possible to maintain stability and functionality. For resection of some masses located in a special position, however, division of the sternoclavicular junction and even partial or near complete resection of the clavicle or the first and second rib can become necessary. Most of these approaches have been developed for treating anterior types of Pancoast's tumors, but they can be applied for resection of some cervicomediastinal masses also.

It is, however, equally crucial to preserve the function of the important nerve structures such as the phrenic, the vagal, and the recurrent

laryngeal nerve. For this reason, and especially for resection of huge and bilaterally extending masses, an approach combining bilateral access to the thoracic cavity together with wide upwards–downwards extension from the neck to the mediastinum, such as the inverse T incision, can become necessary.

If, however, despite optimal exposure, the division of nerves is necessary to achieve a radical resection, it is important to take appropriate concomitant measures to avoid complications. If unilateral resection of a phrenic nerve is required, an additional diaphragmatic plication is usually necessary to avoid an elevated diaphragm leading to lung atelectases because of the reduced intrathoracic volume. After unilateral resection of the recurrent laryngeal nerve, accompanying surgical measures are not mandatory. Especially in reoperations, one might be faced with the situation that a unilateral paralysis of the recurrent laryngeal nerve is preoperatively present and the contralateral nerve might be at risk because of tumor proximity or infiltration. In such cases, a preoperative laser resection of the vocal process might be helpful to enlarge the glottis.

After having the optimal access for tumor resection, an adequate closure of the surgical wound is equally important. Especially after extended resections or in cases of skin impairments after radiotherapy, a primary closure of the wound might not be possible. In such cases, a plastic wound closure with pediculated or free myocutaneous flaps can be necessary. It is important to integrate the potential necessity for plastic wound closure in the planning of the operative strategy.

ANTERIOR APPROACHES
Median Sternotomy

The standard approach to the mediastinum is the median sternotomy. This incision provides excellent access to the anterior and middle compartments and can be extended to the cervical region either by a linear or a curvilinear necklace incision. In this way it becomes suitable for management of combined cervicomediastinal problems. Advantages of such an approach include the sparing of muscles and relatively low postoperative pain. Limitations are a restricted approach to the lateral and posterior aspects of both chest cavities and the risk for sternal infections.

Hemi-Clamshell Incision

The hemi-clamshell incision consists of a combination of an upper partial median sternotomy together with an anterior thoracotomy, usually performed in the second to fifth intercostal space depending on the location of the target area. By this approach, the clavicle must not be divided, and the sternoclavicular joint is left intact, which diminishes postoperative discomfort and improves shoulder stability and appearance. The procedure was proposed as a possible alternative to other transclavicular approaches in patients who suffer from anterior cervicothoracic tumors or for managing injuries to the subclavian vessels.[4] In addition, the vertical part of the incision can be prolonged to the neck along the anterior border of the sternocleidomastoid muscle if this is required. Examples for such a procedure are given in **Fig. 1**.

A paper by Korst and colleagues[1] analyzed the results of this procedure in 42 patients and reported excellent exposure of the pulmonary vessels at the hilum, which facilitated the performance of major anatomic pulmonary resections. No limitations on the extent of additional chest wall resections were found, and the authors concluded that the hemi-clamshell approach is far better than any other described technique for performing of mediastinal lymph node dissection. The only limitation of the hemi-clamshell approach in the resection of tumors of the cervicothoracic

junction is the inadequate exposure of the posterior chest wall and of the neural foramina. This problem is shared with all other anterior approaches to the mediastinum.[1]

The findings of this publication are supported by other papers also,[5] which concluded that the hemi-clamshell incision offers improved exposure to the upper mediastinum and the cervical region, without causing more postoperative morbidity, chest wall complaints, shoulder girdle dysfunction or impairment of pulmonary function than standard approaches.

Inverse T Incision

Only recently, a further extension of the -hemi-clamshell incision, the so-called inverse T incision, has been described, which consists of a full clamshell incision together with a partial upper median sternotomy.[6] This approach provides excellent access to the upper mediastinum, and to both pulmonary hili; it thus allows an effective dissection of virtually the entire upper third of the thoracic cavity. Complete control of both phrenic nerves throughout their whole intrathoracic course is given. Furthermore, the incision can be

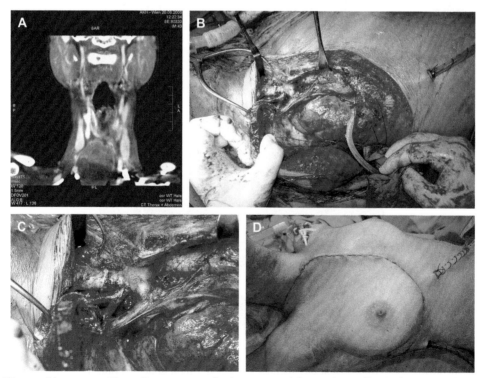

Fig. 1. 27-year-old woman with a solitary neuroendocrine tumor of the cervicomediastinal junction after full preoperative radiochemotherapy. (*A*) Preoperative CT scan showing the large tumor with displacement of the main vessels. (*B*) Intraoperative view after right hemi-clamshell incision with cervical extension. (*C*) Detail of the operative site showing the excellent exposure of the main structures of the cervicothoracic junction. (*D*) Operative site after complete wound closure.

extended easily to the cervical region to allow almost unlimited exposure of cervicothoracic masses. An example of such a procedure is given in **Fig. 2**.

Despite the magnitude of the incision, the stability and functionality of the sternocostal arch are preserved, facilitating a surprisingly fast recovery and a rapid postoperative respiratory rehabilitation. Even though this approach will remain limited to very selected patients, it adds a true alternative to the various more established incisions.

Anterior Cervicothoracic Transclavicular Approach

This approach, developed for the resection of Pancoast tumors invading the thoracic inlet, has been described by Dartevelle and colleagues.[7] Through a large L-shaped anterior cervical incision (**Fig. 3**), the medial half of the clavicle is removed. This allows for dissection or resection of the subclavian vein, sectioning of the anterior scalenus muscle and resection of the cervical portion of the phrenic

nerve if invaded. Furthermore, exposure of the subclavian and vertebral arteries is gained, and dissection of the brachial plexus up to the spinal foramen can be performed. Resection of invaded ribs and en bloc removal of chest wall and lung tumors, either directly or through an extension of the cervical incision into the delto–pectoral groove, can be achieved.

Because the approach is combined with considerable morbidity and focuses anatomically more on lateral parts of the cervicothoracic junction, its use for cervicomediastinal problems remains limited.

Transmanubrial Osteomuscular-Sparing Approach

This approach is a variation of the previously described Dartevelle approach. The technique, previously described,[8] consists of an L-shaped skin incision along the anterior edge of the sternomastoid muscle and two fingers below the clavicle. Insertions of the sternocleidomastoid and

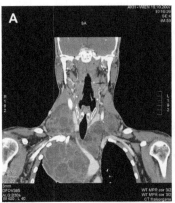
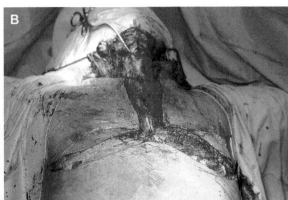
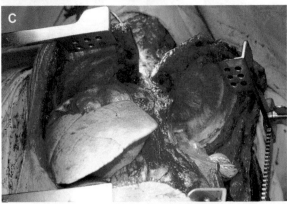

Fig. 2. Preoperative CT scan of a 29-year-old man with extensive lymph node metastases of a germ cell tumor in the cervical and upper thoracic region. The patient was treated in a multidisciplinary way with full induction therapy. Because of the great extent of the involved nodes, an inverse T incision with cervical extension was chosen as approach (A) showing the preoperative CT scan with tumor masses in the anterior and posterior mediastinum extending into the cervical region. (B) Inverse T incision combined with an extended necklace incision for removal of cervicothoracic germ cell tumor masses. (C) Situs after spreading of the sternum and ribs.

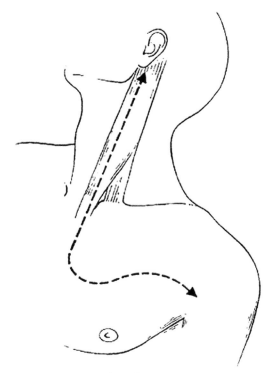

Fig. 3. Anterio-transclavicular approach (Dartevelle).

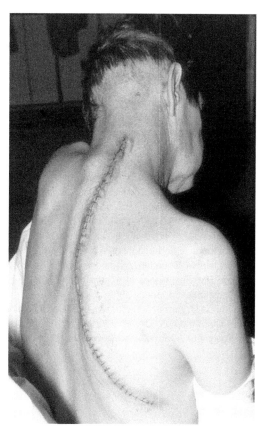

Fig. 4. Paulson approach.

major pectoral muscles on the clavicle are spared. After the division of the internal mammary vessels, an L-shaped section of the manubrium associated with the resection of both the first rib cartilage and the costoclavicular ligament is performed. Thus, an osteomuscular flap containing manubrium edge, clavicle, sternomastoid, and major pectoral muscles is lifted. This provides an excellent exposure of the thoracic in/outlet allowing extended resections. Sparing the main osteomuscular structures, it maintains shoulder mobility by avoiding deformities caused by clavicle resection.[9]

POSTERIOR APPROACHES
Paulson Approach

The high posterior Paulson approach is the standard approach for posterior Pancoast tumors with a posterior thoracotomy extending up to the neck (**Fig. 4**).[10] This approach requires extensive muscle division with frequently prolonged postoperative mobilization and pain. In case of mediastinal tumors, it is reserved for mediastinal masses involving the vertebral column, because virtually all other lesions can be reached by anterior approaches.

SEPARATE APPROACHES

In some rare cases, a cervical incision can be combined with a separate approach through the thorax, either in an open or videothoracoscopic way to achieve radical resection of tumors in the cervicothoracic junction. A combined videothoracoscopic and supraclavicular approach has been described, especially for managing posterior neurogenic tumous.[11] Because in this sensitive area optimal access is required to achieve radical en bloc resection of tumors, these separate approaches will remain limited to highly selected cases.

SUMMARY

Tumors or masses occurring in the cervicothoracic region show a broad variety in their histologic origin. Accordingly, the indication for surgical resection varies, and especially in malignant lesions, surgery frequently is part of a multimodality treatment. Adequate access is important for any operation in a critical region such as the cervicothoracic junction. The anatomic location of the mass to be resected usually dictates either an anterior or posterior approach. The need for appropriate exposure is in addition paralleled by the need to preserve a maximum of important functional structures, to maintain their diligent functional interaction. Careful interdisciplinary preoperative treatment planning is necessary to achieve optimal results.

REFERENCES

1. Korst RJ, Burt ME. Cervicothoracic tumors: results of resection by the hemi-clamshell approach. J Thorac Cardiovasc Surg 1998;115:286–95.
2. Rusch VW. Management of Pancoast tumours. Lancet Oncol 2006;7(12):997–1005.
3. Patterson GA, Cooper JD, Deslauriers J, et al. Pearson's thoracic and esophageal surgery, 3rd edition. Philadelphia: Churchill Livingstone; 2008.
4. Hood RM. Techniques in general thoracic surgery. Philadelphia: Saunders; 1985. p. 64–7.
5. Lardinois D, Sippel M, Gugger M, et al. Morbidity and validity of the hemi-clamshell approach for thoracic surgery. Eur J Cardiothorac Surg 1999;16(2):194–9.
6. Marta GM, Aigner C, Klepetko W. Inverse T incision provides improved accessibility to the upper mediastinum. J Thorac Cardiovasc Surg 2005;129(1):221–3.
7. Dartevelle PG, Chapelier AR, Macchiarini P, et al. Anterior transcervical–thoracic approach for radical resection of lung tumors invading the thoracic inlet. J Thorac Cardiovasc Surg 1993;105(6):1025–34.
8. Grunenwald D, Spaggiari L. Transmanubrial osteomuscular sparing approach for apical chest tumors. Ann Thorac Surg 1997;63:563–6.
9. Spaggiari L, Calabrese L, Gioacchino G, et al. Cervicothoracic tumors resection through transmanubrial osteomuscular sparing. Eur J Cardiothorac Surg 1999;16:564–7.
10. Paulson DL. The importance of defining location and staging of superior pulmonary sulcus tumors. Ann Thorac Surg 1973;15(5):549–51.
11. Yamaguchi M, Yoshino I, Kameyama T, et al. Thoracoscopic surgery combined with a supraclavicular approach for removing a cervicomediastinal neurogenic tumor: a case report. Ann Thorac Cardiovasc Surg 2006;12(3):194–6.

Intraoperative Strategy in Patients with Extended Involvement of Mediastinal Structures

Domenico Massullo, MD*, Pia Di Benedetto, MD,
Giovanni Pinto, MD

KEYWORDS

- Mediastinal tumors • Superior vena cava syndrome
- Airway obstruction • Pericardial effusion • Thymoma

Anesthesia for surgery of mediastinal masses is a challenging procedure, both for adult and pediatric patients. The presence of a mediastinal mass in a patient constantly poses significant anesthesia-related risks, including death. To optimize outcome, clinicians must be able to predict which patients are at highest risk of anesthetic complications. The mediastinum is an area of the body in which a wide range of tissue variability exists; therefore, tumors and cysts that occur in this area can represent many different clinical entities and pathologic processes with different symptoms (**Table 1**). A thorough understanding of the anatomic relationships of the normal structures within the mediastinum is essential in the proper determination of the exact nature of a mass or tumor located in this area and for planning the most appropriate strategy to decrease cardiorespiratory complications in the perioperative period.

PATHOPHYSIOLOGY OF COMPRESSION OF THE TRACHEOBRONCHIAL TREE

Because the maintenance of an airway is a major concern in the perioperative period, the anatomic effect of large mediastinal tumors must be assessed preoperatively to minimize adverse effects.

Awareness and prevention of potential respiratory complications and anticipation of appropriate treatment preparedness are important aspects in the management of these patients. Tracheal and bronchial compression can be evaluated by patient history, physical examination chest radiography, CT scan, MRI, flexible bronchoscopy, and pulmonary function tests.

CT scan accurately assesses the mass volume, the extension and the grade of the tracheobronchial tree compression, and shows the presence of atelectasia, pleural and pericardial effusion, and superior vena cava (SVC) compression.[1,2] King and colleagues[2] correlated preoperative respiratory symptoms with the extent of tracheal compression as measured on CT scan, proposing that these are reasonably accurate indicators of both the significance of the airway compression and the risk of general anesthesia.[3]

Mass-related respiratory collapse can occur in every moment of the perioperative period: when placing the patient in the supine position, at the induction of anesthesia, at extubation, and even a few days after extubation. This kind of complication is a well-recognized complication of general anesthesia in patients with anterior mediastinal masses, with a higher incidence in the pediatric population.[4,5] This risk in the pediatric population

Department of Anesthesiology, University of Rome "La Sapienza", Ospedale S. Andrea, Via di Grottarossa 1035, 00189 Rome, Italy
* Corresponding author.
E-mail address: domenico.massullo@fastwebnet.it (D. Massullo).

Thorac Surg Clin 19 (2009) 113–120
doi:10.1016/j.thorsurg.2008.09.009
1547-4127/08/$ – see front matter © 2009 Published by Elsevier Inc.

Table 1
Sign and symptoms of anterior mediastinal tumors

History	Physical Examination
Cyanosis	Decreased breath sounds
Dyspnea	Wheezing
Orthopnea	Stridor
Cough	Cyanosis

is related to the fact that a mediastinal mass, even a small one, is more likely to have a compressive effect on the small, flexible airway structures and chest cavity of a child.

The induction of general anesthesia in the supine position associated with the use of muscle relaxant leads to a decrease of the dimensions of the rib cage, to a cephalad displacement of the dome of the diaphragm, and to a marked reduction in thoracic volume. This effect is not observed under spontaneous respiration and many patients affected by large tumors may be asymptomatic. A possible explanation is that in the supine position, two opposing forces maintain the position of the mediastinal mass: the negative intrathoracic pressure and the gravity. The first one pulls the mass upward, while the second one pulls it downward in a posterior direction. When the patient lies supine, the gravity becomes dominant and pulls the mass onto tracheobronchial tree or heart. The further reduction of intrathoracic pressure for cessation of spontaneous ventilation, the induction of anesthesia, and the positive ventilation shift the balance of pressure in favor of gravity. Moreover, the pharmacologic muscle relaxation of the smooth bronchial muscles reduces the tone of the tracheobronchial tree and decreases the resistance to the weight of the mass, which therefore increases its compression on the airways.

Another physiologic mechanism related to the transpleural gradient is the increasing diameter of the airways during inspiration: with muscle relaxation and positive-pressure ventilation, a reduction of the diameter of the airways occurs, leading to a total airway-collapse case of critical stenosis (more than 50%).[4,6] When the patient lies supine, inhaled gas is preferentially distributed in the non-dependent lung area, while in the dependent lung, tatelectasis is likely to occur, thus determining a "shunt effect." The association of the shunt effect and the critically restricted airways causes a rapid falling in arterial oxygenation.

Usually, under spontaneous breathing, the physiologic laminar flow in the distal bronchi allows for gas diffusion. During controlled artificial ventilation with positive pressure in a reduced airway cross section, there is an increase of gas-molecular acceleration and a consequent turbulent poststenotic flow that decreases the gas diffusion in the small areas. This results in a decreased gas exchange and arterial vein mismatching, shunting formation, impaired expiration, increased airway resistence, air-trapping phenomenon, and as a final result, severe hypoxemia. However, the impairment of respiration because of the compression of the anterior mediastinal mass on respiratory fuction may be unknown and it may elude all static diagnostic tests, as it is a dynamic, intermittent phenomenon.[4]

Whenever possible, especially in symptomatic children in which this problem can be anticipated, after the induction of anesthesia spontaneous ventilation should be continued, avoiding muscle relaxation and positive-pressure ventilation. Compared with adults, children are much more often symptomatic and their respiratory function can be rapidly complicated by emergencies. Factors for increased morbidity are a smaller thoracic cage, less pulmonary reserve, and a more frail cartilaginous structure of the airway. Small decreases in diameter produce relatively larger decreases in luminal area and increases in airway resistance.[7] If the procedure has to be conducted in controlled, positive ventilation, both left-lateral and prone positions can minimize the compression on mediastinal structures.[8,9]

Another mechanism involved in the increase of mass compression on mediastinal organs is the increase of the venous return in the supine position. This blood overload increases the mass volume and its compression on adjacent structures. It is important to point out that, in children, the incidence of anesthesia-related life-threatening respiratory complications, according to many investigators, is as high as 20%.[10,11] Azarow and colleagues[12] compared the mortality and morbidity in the adult and pediatric population and found no statistical difference between the two groups. However, mortality associated with perioperative respiratory complications is higher in pediatric patients.[13] This result is because of the different causes of mortality in the two groups; death in children can be attribuited mainly to perioperative respiratory complications, whereas in adults death is mainly because of uncontrolled malignancy.

In the adult population, respiratory complications are unusual, and in the literature there is no single case report about such complications. This means that in the adult, asymptomatic patient, general anesthesia can be induced safely, if the preoperative radiologic and bronchoscopic findings do not show the presence of an exceedingly large compressing mass. The pathophysiologic impairment of the tracheobronchial tree should suggest when it is possible to use loco-regional techniques in cooperative children or in adults.[3,14,15] In small infants or newborns, these techniques, associated with light general anesthesia and spontaneous breathing, are feasible both for intraoperative and postoperative management.

PATHOPHYSIOLOGY OF COMPRESSION OF THE HEART AND GREAT VESSELS

The derailment of hemodynamic parameters occurs when mediastinal masses infiltrate or surround the SVC, pulmonary artery, or heart. However, because of the immediate proximity of the mediastinal structures, cardiovascular and respiratory effects are combined in most cases.[16]

Compression of the pulmonary artery is relatively rare; its contiguity with the aorta and tracheobronchial tree offers a certain protection against mechanical compression.[17] Reduction in the diameter of the pulmonary trunk or one of the main pulmonary arteries, with consecutive impairment of perfusion, can cause hypoxemia, hypotension, or cardiocirculatory arrest.[18] This is the expression of serious, acute overload of the right heart and reduced preload of the left ventricle. The patient is usually asymptomatic and the most important symptom is syncope during a forced Valsalva maneuver.[19]

Hemodynamic imbalance occurs if the pulmonary artery blood flow declines below the critical limit. Triggering factors may be the induction of general anesthesia, the supine position on the operating table, the administration of muscle relaxants, and positive-pressure ventilation . When suspicion of pulmonary artery compression arises, there are no determinants as to which patient will be intolerant to general anesthesia. A primed pump for extracorporeal membrane oxygenation and a prepared team should thus be immediately available in the operating room.[20,21] However, the use of cardiopulmonary bypass as a rescue maneuver is unrealistic. The patient could suffer neurologic complications because of the time needed to cannulate and restore sufficient blood circulation and oxygenation.[22] Femoro-femoral cardiopulmonary bypass can be instituted before induction of general anesthesia.[23] Compression of the airways and the venous system in the antero-superior mediastinum leads to superior vena cava syndrome (SVCS) (**Table 2**). The SVC is particularly vulnerable to extrinsic compression. This is because of the low intravascular pressure, the thin vessel wall, and the neighborhood of solid structures as lymph nodes and bronchi. The low intravascular pressure also represents a risk factor for thrombus formation,

---

Table 2
Symptoms of tracheobronchial and cardiovascular structures compression

Compression of tracheobronchial tree	Orthopnea Rest and stress dyspnea Dyspnea, especially in the supine or on the side Inspiratory and exspiratory stridor Recurrent bronchities Cough
Compression of pulmonary artery and heart	Cyanosis (especially in the supine) Dizziness, syncope (especially in the supine and in Valsalva maneuver) Orthopnea, dyspnea Pallor (sudden change of body position) Pulsus paradoxus Blood pressure fluctuations
Compression of superior vena cava	Cyanosis Face, neck, chest, limb edema Papilledema Periorbital edema Breast edema (similar to gynecomastia) Larynxedema (inspiratory stridor, dyspnea) Jugular, arm, thoracic venous dilatation (no veins collapse while lifting the arm upon heart level) Hypotension Syncope Dysphagia Central symptoms: headache, awareness disturbance, nausea, vomiting, neurologic failure

especially in association with indwelling catheters. The impaired venous drainage from the head and neck reduces preload of the right ventricle, causes reduction of cardiac output, and increases central venous pressure, which results in interstitial edema and retrograde collateral flow.[17]

The rapidity of the obstruction and its location causes the severity of the syndrome. The most common localization of the compression is the right chest side (4:1) above the confluence of azygos vein. In this case, the azygos venous system is dilated to accept the shunted blood, with higher venous pressure flowing from the upper body. If the obstruction is below the confluence of the azygos vein, the blood flows to the inferior vena cava and the heart through the upper abdominal veins, requiring higher venous pressure.[24] SVCS causes remarkable problems in the anesthetic management.

Venous congestion can cause severe laryngeal edema, acute airway obstruction, and airway difficulties during induction or emergence from anesthesia. Surgery should be performed with the patient in the Fowler position.[25] Fluid administration should be careful: excessive fluid may increase venous pressure in the upper body, while a decrease in the preload, leading to hypotension in association with compromised venous return, is equally undesirable. Because the SVC circulation is compromised, fluids and drugs should to be administered through the inferior vena cava circulation, preferably via the femoral vein. The obstruction also compromises the cerebral venous drainage and hyperhydratation can cause cerebral edema. An important surgical problem is intraoperative bleeding associated with high central venous pressure.

Large mediastinal masses may also directly involve the heart. Direct myocardial infiltration is a rare event. Pericardial involvement can cause cardiovascular effects that are similar to pericardial tamponade or constrictive pericarditis.[26] Arrhythmias or a low cardiac output syndrome are frequently observed.[27] Johnson and colleagues[28] suggest that the decrease in cardiac index results from an increase in right ventricular afterload caused by right ventricular outflow tract obstruction, pericardial effusion, or SVC obstruction or a combination of these factors. The aorta is usually spared from involvement because of its location, thick muscular walls, and high intraluminal pressure. Cardiovascular changes described above can amplify the depression of myocardial function and increase the risk of death upon induction of anesthesia.[29]

PREOPERATIVE ASSESSMENT

The intraoperative strategy is determined preoperatively and starts with the anesthesiologic assessment. The likelihood of malignancy is influenced primarily by the following three factors: mass location, patient age, and the presence or absence of symptoms. Although more than two-thirds of mediastinal tumors are benign, masses in the anterior compartment are more likely to be malignant.[14]

The stratification of the perioperative risk is based on the analysis of patient health status, the associated comorbidities, and the cardio-respiratory function. It is therefore important to asses the mass localization, its extension, and the grade of compression of the intrathoracic structures, such as the trachea and great vessels, the SVC, and the pulmonary artery, as well as the lungs and the heart. Respiratory function can be assessed with blood-gas analysis, flexible bronchoscopy, and pulmonary function tests. Data of postural spirometry in upright and in supine position are not related with perioperative respiratory complications.[30]

Cardiac reserve is assessed by EKG, echocardiography, and CT-scan. Echocardiography further investigates cardiac function as related to the degree of obstruction of right ventricular outflow tract and pulmonary artery, right ventricle dimensions, presence of pericardial effusions, and infiltration. The radiologic findings (CT or thoracic X-ray) can show the grade and kind of compression of the main mediastinal organs.

From an anesthesiologic standpoint, another important consideration is the kind of surgery required; it is quite obvious that the anesthesiologic conduct is greatly different if either single biopsy or extended resection is planned. Expected postoperative pain is also different. In those patients who require extended surgery, accurate postoperative analgesia has to be planned for its beneficial effect on the patient's outcome and rapid recovery. Other factors may influence the patient outcome and they depend not only on the American Society of Anesthesiologists status, but also by the kind of surgery and the surgeon's skill.

Intraoperative strategy for blood transfusion has to be carefully planned and, whenever possible, autologous blood has to be collected preoperatively in all benign lesions in addition to intraoperative blood salvage. Before surgery it could be useful to stimulate the bone marrow to produce red blood cells with preoperative administration of iron, B vitamin, or erithropoyetin.

It is important that any patient with a mediastinal mass is thoroughly assessed by the anesthesiologist in case concomitant surgery is needed. Locoregional anesthesia should be preferred whenever is possible to prevent airway compression, or alternatively the mediastinal mass should be treated beforehand.

In the postoperative period it is mandatory to recover the operated patient in the intensive care unit. After the risk stratification is completed, it is necessary to openly discuss these issues with the patient and to explain the kind and intensity of postoperative pain.

OPERATIVE PROCEDURES

Based on the preoperative condition, the patient has to be transferred to the operating room fully monitored and under direct physician surveillance. In cases of severe dyspnoea, the patient is placed in the sitting position on the operative bed. After his or her arrival in the operating room, a large bore cannula vein has to be placed. If the patient has SVCS, the preferred site to place the central venous access is the femoral vein, possibly under ultrasound guidance. Invasive monitorization of arterial blood pressure via radial artery is also mandatory.

Whenever it is possible, before the induction of anesthesia and in the absence of specific contraindications, such as congenital or acquired coagulopathy, anticoagulant or antiaggregant theraphy, patient's refusal, sepsis, or local infection, a thoracic epidural catheter has to be placed.[31,32] This technique is defined as the "gold standard for postoperative analgesia."[33] Postoperatively, the infusion of analgesic solution (local anesthetic alone or in combination with adjuvants) can be administered with different modalities: continuous epidural or controlled patient for at least 72 hours.

Alternatively, another feasible locoregional technique is the continuous thoracic paravertebral blockade, fielding unilateral dermatomal anesthesia.[34,35] The resultant blockade can be regarded as an ipsilateral continuous thoracic epidural, except that there are no significant hemodynamic changes nor major complications, such as epidural ematoma.[36] The paravertebral catheter is ideally inserted one to two segmental levels below the thoracotomy incision line. Pain from sternotomy can be effectively relieved by two paravertebral catheters at the bilateral D_6 to D_7 level.[37] Even in this technique, the analgesic solution can be infused for several days.

For all patients with severe tracheobronchial compression, it is safer to avoid premedication and it is necessary to predispose all material for awake intubation, either via flexible or rigid bronchoscopy.[38] To improve patient safety, two skilled anesthetists have to be present, as well as a surgeon experienced with the use of rigid bronchoscopy. Rigid bronchoscopy may be necessary to overcome airway stenosis when the mass compresses the tracheobronchial tree distally to the tip of the tube.

For awake fiberoptic broncoscopic intubation, the hypopharynx and the glottis are anesthetized with topic to attenuate the pharyngolaryngeal reflex during bronchoscopy. Mild sedation can be administered with 0.07-mg/kg midazolam or 0.025-mcg/kg to 0.1-mcg/kg per minute of remifentanil. The use of short-life drugs with the possibility of rapid recovery from general anesthesia with the return of normal muscle tone and spontaneous breathing is recommended.[39,40] The ultrashort remifentanil opiod allows a mitigation of cough for its specific action on bronchial cough reflex receptors.[41]

The better position for intubating is the sitting position (Fowler position),[42] after a preoxygenation with O_2 100%. The endotracheal tube used should have a maximum inside diameter and high resistance to extrinsic compression (eg, spiral tube). According to the kind of surgical procedure, particularly in adults, the placement of a double-lumen tube could be necessary. In children, to ensure one-lung ventilation, instead of the double-lumen tube the authors' preference goes to the a bronchial blocker placed with the aid of a pediatric flexible bronchoscope.

With a large mass within the thorax, the positive-pressure ventilation can exacerbate the compression of the tracheabronchial tree. Assisted positive-pressure ventilation should first be gradually taken over manually, to assure that positive-pressure ventilation is possible, and only in that case should a short-acting muscle relaxant be administered.

If positive-pressure ventilation causes a fall in arterial oxygenation, then a change in the patient position should be considered, lateral or prone, to shift the compressive mass to other intrathoracic districts.[43] After proper positioning of the endotracheal tube, and appropriate check of the trachea and main bronchi through bronchoscope, anesthtic drugs for both narcosis and analgesia have to be administered. The short acting opioid remifentanil seems to be particularly suitable for this kind of surgical procedure and it has to be delivered in continous infusion with different modalities, either as total intravenous anesthesia or target-controlled infusion (TCI). Both techniques allow for rapid washout from receptorial sites after the end of administration, thus decreasing the risk of postoperative respiratory narcotic depression. When the surgical procedure does not need full muscle relaxation, ventilation should be performed under spontaneous breathing.

For the patients in whom the compression of the mass exerts its effect mainly on the superior vena cava, the degree of cardiovascular compromise guides to the conduct of the anesthesiologic intraoperative monitoring. As previously described, a compression of the pulmonary artery can occur immediately before the induction of anesthesia. The loss of negative intrathoracic pressure combined with the supine position may cause a rapid compression of the pulmonary artery, leading to a rapid decrease of oxygen blood saturation, hypotension, and even to fatal cardiac arrest.[16,44,45] In these circumstances, the changing of position (lateral or prone) can restore circulation.

In all cases in which the compression of the mass impairs the venous drainage from the upper part of the body, the right ventricular failure is directly related to the severity of the SVCS. To avoid the detrimental effect of loss of heat, the core temperature has to be measured through a tympanic or esophageal probe, and a heating system both for intravenous fluids and for the body should be available.[46,47]

First-line intraoperative devices for hemodynamic monitoring are EKG-5 electrodes, end-tidal capnography, invasive A-line, central venous pressure monitoring (via the femoral vein in severe SVCS), and transoesophageal echocardiography.[48,49] Second-line monitoring include Swan Ganz catheter to evidence the wedge pressure and cardiac output useful to appropriately administer fluids, and the INVOS Cerebral Oximeter system, which monitors the critical balance between oxygen delivery and cerebral consumption.[50,51]

The Bispectral Index is useful to tailor the patient's dose of delivered anesthetic drugs.[52] This device can analyze the effects of anesthesia on a patient's level of consciousness by measuring the brain activity. This allows a reduction of an unnecessary amount of anesthetic drugs with decreased hemodynamic impairment, especially when they are administered with an open TCI system (closed loop anesthesia).[53,54] With this infusional modality, the most suitable opioid for intraoperative TCI infusion is remifentanil, with an effect site target ranging from 3-ng mL^{-1} to 5-ng mL^{-1}. The latter is employed in combination with a continuous TCI infusion (Schnider model) of propofol, ranging from 3.5-ng mL^{-1} to 7.0-ng mL^{-1} at the plasma or effector site.[55]

In severe SVCS it is necessary to keep ready vasoactive drugs such as phenilylnephrine or noradrenaline, which can restore systemic blood pressure, implementing systemic vascular resistance when cardiovascular collapse occurs. The attempt to treat hypotension solely by rapid infusion of fluids to increase intravascular volume is unlikely to be successful.[26] During surgical resection of mediastinal masses, a massive hemorrhage may occur, and

all appropriate measures to enable rapid replacement of blood during the intervention must taken.

Mediastinal tumors can surround or infiltrate phrenic or recurrent laringeal nerves.[56,57] The resection of these nerves during surgery can cause serious respiratory problems during the postoperative period. During particularly demanding surgical procedures, extracorporeal membrane oxygenation should be considered as an option.[58,59] This occurs rarely in an emergency intraoperative setting, but rather as a carefully planned rescue technique.[60] As previously mentioned, the femoral vein can be cannulated in local anesthesia before induction of general anesthesia.

To improve the postoperative analgesia, in adults 30 minutes before the disconnection of remifentanil infusion, 10-mg morphine sulfate has to be administered intravenously, and after the recovery from anesthesia 1-mg/ml morphine every 5 to 7 minutes has to be titrated according to the patient visual analog pain score (VAS) and then stopped when the VAS reaches the value of 3.[61]

According to current guidelines, multimodal analgesia with the combined use of opiates, paracetamol, and nonsteroidal anti-inflammatory drugs as a dose-rescue to reduce the amount of a single analgesic and their side effects should be provided.[62,63] The most appropriate modality for postoperative opioid administration is the patient-controlled analgesia technique, which requires a fully awake and cooperative patient.[64,65]

In conclusion, patients with mediastinal masses have specific problems that need careful evaluation before surgery because any invasive procedure is associated with a high risk of morbidity and mortality. Life threatening complications, such as respiratory or cardiovascular failure, may occur at any moment during the perioperative period. A multidisciplinary approach represents the most important factor to ensure a successful outcome and the operative team must be experienced in the management of these patients.

REFERENCES

1. King DR, Patrick LE, Ginn-Pease ME, et al. Pulmonary function is compromised in children with mediastinal lymphoma. J Pediatr Surg 1997;32:294–9.

2. Shamberger RC, Holzman RS, Griscom NT, et al. Prospective evaluation by computed tomography and pulmonary function tests of children with mediastinal masses. Surgery 1995;118:468–71.

3. Anghelescu DL, Burgoyne LL, Liu T, et al. Clinical and diagnostic imaging findings predict anesthetic complications in children presenting with malignant mediastinal masses. Pediatr Anaesth 2007;17(11): 1090–8.

4. Narang S, Harte BH. Body SC. Anesthesia for patients with a mediastinal mass. Anesthesiol Clin North America 2001;19(3):559–79.

5. Shamberger RC. Preanesthetic evaluation of children with anterior mediastinal masses. Semin Pediatr Surg 1999;8(2):61–8.

6. Shamberger RC, Holzman RS, Griscom NT, et al. CT quantitation of tracheal cross-sectional area as a guide to the surgical and anesthetic management of children with anterior mediastinal masses. J Pediatr Surg 1991;26:138–42.

7. Azizkhan RG, Dudgeon DL, Buck JR, et al. Life-threatening airway obstruction as a complication to the management of mediastinal masses in children. J Pediatr Surg 1985;20:816–22.

8. Gothard JW. Anesthetic considerations for patients with anterior mediastinal masses. Anesth Clin 2008;26(2):305–14.

9. Sibert KS, Biondi JW, Hirsch NP. Spontaneous respiration during thoracotomy in a patient with a mediastinal mass. Anesth Analg 1987;66:904–7.

10. Piro AJ, Weiss DR, Hellman S. Mediastinal Hodgkin's disease: a possible danger for intubation anesthesia. Int J Radiat Oncol Biol Phys 1976;1:415–9.

11. Ferrari LR, Bedford RF. General anesthesia prior to treatment of anterior mediastinal masses in pediatric cancer patients. Anesthesiology 1990;72:991–5.

12. Azarow KS, Pearl RH, Zurcher R, et al. Primary mediastinal masses: A comparison of adult and pediatric populations. J Thorac Cardiovasc Surg 1993;106:67–72.

13. Victory RA, Casey W, Doherty P, et al. Cardiac and respiratory complications of mediastinal lymphomas. Anaesth Intens Care 1993;21:366–9.

14. Strollo DC, Rosado-de-Christenson ML, Jett JR. Primary mediastinal tumors: Part 1 Tumors of the anterior mediastinum. Chest 1997;112:511–22.

15. Rendina EA, Venuta F, De Giacomo T, et al. Coloni GF Biopsy of anterior mediastinal masses under local anesthesia. Ann Thorac Surg 2002;74(5):1720–2 [discussion: 1722–3].

16. Cheung SL, Lerman J. Mediastinal masses and anesthesia in children. Anesth Clin North America 1998;16:893–911.

17. Miller RD. Anesthesia. 4th edition. Edinburgh (UK): Churchill Livingstone; (1994). p. 1737–9.

18. Levin H, Bursztein S, Heifetz M. Cardiac arrest in a child with a mediastinal mass. Anesth Analg 1985;64:1129–30.

19. Froese AB, Bryan AC. Effects of anesthesia and paralysis on diaphragmatic mechanics in man. Anesthesiology 1974;41:242–55.

20. Hall KD, Friedman M. Extracorporeal oxygenation for induction of anesthesia in a patient with an intrathoracic tumor. Anesthesiology 1975;42:493–5.

21. Pullerits J, Holzman R. Anaesthesia for patients with mediastinal masses. Can J Anaesth 1989;36(6):681–8.

22. Takeda S, Shinichiro M, Omori K, et al. Surgical rescue for life-threatening hypoxemia caused by a mediastinal tumor. Ann Thorac Surg 1999;68:2324–6.

23. Tempe DK, Arya R, Dubey S. Mediastinal mass resection: femorofemoral cardiopulmonary bypass before induction of anesthesia in the management of airway obstruction. J Cardiothorac Vasc Anesth 2001;15(2):233–6.

24. Yellin A, Rosen A, Reichert N, et al. Superior vena cava syndrome: the myth-the facts. Am Rev Respir Dis 1990;141(5):1114–8.

25. Neuman GG, Weingarten AE, Abramowitz RM, et al. The anesthetic management of the patient with an anterior mediastinal mass. Anesthesiology 1984;60(2):144–7.

26. Canedo MI, Otken L, Stefadouros MA. Echocardiographic features of cardiac compression by a thymoma simulating cardiac tamponade and obstruction of the superior vena cava. Br Heart J 1977;39:1038–42.

27. Mackie AM, Watson CB. Anaesthesia and mediastinal masses. A case report and review of the literature. Anaesthesia 1984;39:899–903.

28. Johnson D, Hurst T, Cujec B, et al. Cardiopulmonary effects of an anterior mediastinal mass in dogs anesthetized with halothane. Anesthesiology 1991;74(4):725–36.

29. Keon TP. Death on induction of anesthesia for cervical node biopsy. Anesthesiology 1981;55:471–2.

30. Hatniuk OW, Corcoran PC, Sierra A. Spirometry in surgery for anterior mediastinal masses. Chest 2001;120(4):1152–6.

31. Loran MS, Emasd BM. Thoracic epidural catheter in the management of a child with an anterior mediastinal mass: a case report and literature review. Paediatr Anaesth 2006;16(2):200–5.

32. Buvanendran A, Mohajer P, Pombar X, et al. Perioperative management with epidural anesthesia for a parturient with superior vena caval obstruction. Anesth Analg 2004;98(4):1160–3.

33. Nimmo SM. Benefit and outcome after epidural analgesia. Continuing Education in Anaesthesia Critical Care and Pain 2004;4(2):44–7.

34. Davies RG, Myles PS, Graham JM. A comparison of the analgesic efficacy and side-effects of paravertebral vs epidural blockade for thoracotomy—a systematic review and meta-analysis of randomized trials. Br J Anaesth 2006;96(4):418–26.

35. Hammer GB. Pediatric thoracic anesthesia. Anesth Analg 2001;92:1449–64.

36. Ruppen W, Derry S, McQuay HJ, et al. Incidence of epidural haematoma and neurological injury in cardiovascular patients with epidural analgesia/anaesthesia: systematic review and meta-analysis. BMC Anesthesiol 2006;6:10.

37. Cantó M, Sánchez MJ, Casas MA, et al. Bilateral paravertebral blockade for conventional cardiac surgery. Anaesthesia 2003;58(4):365–70.

38. Capdeville M. The management of a patient with tracheal compression undergoing combined resection of an anterior mediastinal mass and aortic valve replacement with coronary artery bypass graft surgery: utility of the laryngeal mask airway and Aintree intubation catheter. J Cardiothorac Vasc Anesth 2007;21(2):259–61.

39. Machata AM, Gonano C, Holzer A, et al. Awake nasotracheal fiberoptic intubation: patient comfort, intubating conditions, and hemodynamic stability during conscious sedation with remifentanil. Anesth Analg 2003;97(3):904–8.

40. Puchner W, Egger P, Pühringer F, et al. Evaluation of remifentanil as single drug for awake fiberoptic intubation. Acta Anaesthesiol Scand 2002;46(4):350–4.

41. Hohlrieder M, Tiefenthaler W, Klaus H, et al. Effect of total intravenous anaesthesia and balanced anaesthesia on the frequency of coughing during emergence from the anaesthesia. Br J Anaesth 2007; 99(4):587–91.

42. Prakash UB, Abel MD, Hubmayr RD. Mediastinal mass and tracheal obstruction during general anesthesia. Mayo Clin Proc 1988;63(10):1004–11.

43. Vas L, Nalguni F, Naik V. Case report. Anaesthetic management of an infant with anterior mediastinal mass. Pediatr Anaesth 1999;9:439–43.

44. Yamashita M, Chin I, Horigome H, et al. Sudden fatal cardiac arrest in a child with an unrecognized anterior mediastinal mass. Resuscitation 1990;19(2):175–7.

45. Somers GR, Smith CR, Perrin DG, et al. Sudden unexpected death in infancy and childhood due to undiagnosed neoplasia: An autopsy study. Am J Forensic Med Pathol 2006;27(1):64–9.

46. Insler SR, Sessler DI. Perioperative thermoregulation and temperature monitoring. Anesthesiol Clin 2006; 24(4):823–37.

47. Putzu M, Casati A, Berti M, et al. Clinical complications, monitoring and management of perioperative mild hypothermia: anesthesiological features. Acta Biomed 2007;78(3):163–9.

48. Tee EA, Shah PM. Transesophageal echocardiography. J Intensive Care Med 1992;7(3):113–26 [review].

49. Ding ZP, Quek SS, Chee TS. Transoesophageal echocardiography—an overview. Ann Acad Med Singapore 1990;19(1):99–103.

50. Nollert G, Mohnle P, Tassani-Prell P, et al. Determinants of cerebral oxygenation during cardiac surgery. Circulation 1995;92:II327–33.

51. Taillefer MC, Denault AY. Cerebral near-infrared spectroscopy in adult heart surgery: systematic review of its clinical efficacy. Can J Anesth 2005;52:79–87.

52. Halliburton JR, McCarthy EJ. Perioperative monitoring with the electroencephalogram and the Bispectral Index monitor. AANA J 2000;68(4):333–40.

53. Liu N, Chazot T, Trillat B, et al. Closed-loop titration of propofol guided by the Bispectral Index. Ann Fr Anesth Reanim 2007;26(10):850–4 [Epub 2007 Aug 14].

54. Yamamoto S, Goto K, Yasuda N, et al. Cardiac anesthesia induction by low target plasma concentration setting of propofol using target-controlled infusion. Masui 2008;57(6):691–5.

55. Macquaire V, Cantraine F, Schmartz D, et al. Target-controlled infusion of propofol induction with or without plasma concentration constraint in high-risk adult patients undergoing cardiac surgery. Acta Anaesthesiol Scand 2002;46(8): 1010–6.

56. Elefteriades J, Singh M, Tang P, et al. Unilateral diaphragm paralysis: etiology, impact, and natural history. J Cardiovasc Surg (Torino) 2008;49(2): 289–95.

57. Shirakusa T, Tsutsui M, Montonaga, et al. Intrathoracic tumors arising from the vagus nerve. Review of resected tumors in Japan. Scand J Thorac Cardiovasc Surg 1989;23(2):173–5.

58. John RE, Narang VPS. A boy with an anterior mediastinal mass. Anaesthesia 1988;43:864–6.

59. Hensley FA. A practical approach to cardiac anesthesia. 3rd edition. Philadelphia: Lippincott Williams & Wilkins; 2003. p. 672–4.

60. Slinger P, Karli C. Management of the patient with a large anterior mediastinal mass: recurring myths. Current Opin Anaesth 2007;20(1):1–3.

61. Aubrun F, Valade N, Riou B. Intravenous morphine titration. Ann Fr Anesth Reanim 2004;23(10): 973–85.

62. Kruger M, McRae K. Pain management in cardiothoracic practice. Surg Clin North Am 1999;79(2): 387–400 [review].

63. Roediger L, Larbuisson R, Lamy M. New approaches and old controversies to postoperative pain control following cardiac surgery. Eur J Anaesthesiol 2006;23(7):539–50.

64. Marret E, Bazelly B, Taylor G, et al. Paravertebral block with ropivacaine 0.5% versus systemic analgesia for pain relief after thoracotomy. Ann Thorac Surg 2005;79(6):2109–13.

65. Pettersson PH, Lindskog EA, Owall A. Patient-controlled versus nurse-controlled pain treatment after coronary artery bypass surgery. Acta Anaesthesiol Scand 2000;44(1):43–7.

The Role of Surgery in Recurrent Thymic Tumors

Enrico Ruffini, MD*, Pier Luigi Filosso, MD, Alberto Oliaro, MD

KEYWORDS

- Thymic tumors • Mediastinal neoplasms
- Salvage surgery • Thymoma • Recurrence

Mediastinal tumors include various malignancies arising from structures anatomically located in this area and from adjacent organs. Optimal management depends upon histology that usually is obtained through mediastinal biopsy. Treatment options are chemotherapy, radiotherapy, and surgery alone or in combination.

Although the role of surgery in the treatment of most mediastinal malignancies is well-established, either alone or as part of a combined modality treatment, far less clear is the value of surgical resection for recurrent or chemorefractory mediastinal tumors.

Because of the rarity of mediastinal tumors, most of the suggestions proposed by the authors about the role of salvage surgery or surgery for recurrent neoplasms are based more upon the surgeons' personal experience and individualized treatment than upon an evidence-based method. Also, most series concerning surgery for recurrent mediastinal tumors suffer from a selection bias; in fact, the fittest patients usually are offered surgery, with an anticipated survival advantage in the surgical group.

Nonetheless, even if the aforementioned issues are taken into consideration, a role for surgery in recurrent mediastinal tumors, and in particular for thymoma, is undisputable.

THYMOMA

Thymoma is the most common mediastinal neoplasm in adults, representing 50% of the tumors of the anterior mediastinum.[1] Despite its indolent behavior, thymomas should be considered malignant because of the potential local invasion, pleural dissemination and, although rare, systemic metastases. Because of its slow-growing tendency, long-term follow-up is needed after resection to detect recurrences and assess prognosis. Recurrence of thymoma is not uncommon, occurring in up to 30% to 50% of the patients after complete resection.[2,3] The pattern of recurrence is highly variable, including local recurrence, pleural implants, and systemic metastases.

Some reports showed a relatively prolonged clinical course after recurrence of thymoma, confirming the somehow slow-growing behavior of the neoplasm.[4,5] For this reason, resection of local recurrence appears appalling, and may allow satisfactory long-term survival rates. Other authors, however, correctly pointed out the selection bias in the surgical series; in fact, surgery usually is offered to the more fit patients with presumably resectable recurrence; this variable clearly limits the interpretation of the results.[5]

PREVALENCE AND PATTERN OF RECURRENCE AFTER RESECTION OF THYMOMA

Recurrence after complete resection of thymoma ranges from 5% to 50% and clearly is related to stage. Capsulated tumors recur very rarely (0% to 5%);[4] invasive tumors show a recurrence rate ranging from 20% to 50% from stage 1 to stage 4a respectively.[1,6] In patients who have initial stage 4a thymoma, however, pleural recurrence should be interpreted carefully, because complete resection is often difficult. Additionally, pleural

Division of Thoracic Surgery, University of Torino, 3 Via Genova, 10126 Torino, Italy
* Corresponding author.
E-mail address: enrico.ruffini@unito.it (E. Ruffini).

Thorac Surg Clin 19 (2009) 121–131
doi:10.1016/j.thorsurg.2008.09.005
1547-4127/08/$ – see front matter © 2009 Published by Elsevier Inc.

relapse by means of pleural implants is extremely frequent.

The site of recurrence includes the mediastinum, lung, pleura, or distant sites. Recurrences confined to the mediastinum are less frequent (30%), while recurrence within the pleura is more frequent, occurring in about 50% of the cases. Pericardial, lung, and other intrathoracic recurrences are rare. Distant metastases represent less than 5% of the cases.[7] Recurrence may occur within the thymus left in place during the first surgical procedure or in the thoracic compartment where thymoma was located, in the pleural space opened to allow complete resection, and even at the site of the wound of the first operation or the mediastinal biopsy initially performed for tissue diagnosis.[8] This behavior may be related to disruption of the capsula during operation. Therefore, complete resection of the entire thymus is recommended, along with extreme care during dissection and en bloc resection of the surrounding structures infiltrated by the tumor. This observation contributes to raise some questions about the appropriateness of resecting small and well-capsulated thymomas by video-assisted thoracic surgery (VATS) or robotic assistance;[9–11] long-term follow-up is required to evaluate safety and efficacy of minimally invasive techniques, and exclude the possibility of an increased risk of pleural recurrence.

The three most important predictors of recurrence after thymoma resection are stage, World Health Organization (WHO) histologic classification, and completeness of resection (**Box 1**).[12–15] Also, involvement of the great vessels and tumor size have been advocated as negative prognostic factors, although they are not accepted universally.[3,16]

Tumor staging is a key factor to predict recurrence. In 1981, Masaoka and colleagues[17] proposed an anatomic/surgical classification based on the presence of gross or microscopic invasion of the capsule or the surrounding intrathoracic structures and the presence of distant metastases. The classification is still effective, with minor revisions adopted in 1994.[18] A useful adjunct to the Masaoka staging system was proposed by Haniuda and colleagues[19] in 1996; he suggested a stratification based on type of involvement of the parietal pleural (pleural factor, p) and pericardium (pericardial factor, c). Macroscopic adhesion to the pleura or pericardium without microscopic invasion was designed as p1 or c1, while microscopic invasion was termed as p2 or c2. All patients who had either adhesion (p1/c1) or microscopic invasion (p2/c2) were at increased risk of recurrence. Postoperative mediastinal irradiation was effective in preventing recurrence in patients who had p1 but not in those who had p2 or c2 tumors. The same author in a subsequent study[5] reported that, although the recurrence rates increased with the clinical stage and p and c factors, these variables did not show any impact on postrecurrence survival.

WHO histologic classification was proposed in 1999[20] and subsequently updated in 2004;[21] it has been found to represent a strong independent predictor of thymoma recurrence. For clinical purpose, some authors[22] suggested to consider four groups: A (A and AB); early B (B1 and B2), B3, and C, with an increasing tendency to local aggressiveness and recurrence. Tumor histology also was found to correlate with stage, because most type A and AB tumors are stage 1–2, while B2/B3 types are more often stage 3–4.

THE ROLE OF ADJUVANT RADIATION THERAPY IN PREVENTING RECURRENCE

Because most thymoma recurrences occur within the mediastinum, several authors have recommended postoperative radiotherapy (RT) to reduce the rate of this complication. Therefore, many centers started to administer radiation therapy in all resected patients;[23–25] however, subsequent reports showed that adjuvant RT was associated with late morbidity to the heart, lungs, and other mediastinal structures.[26–28] Also, the cost of radiation therapy is sometimes higher than surgery. Last, mediastinal radiation does not prevent pleural implants, which represents the most common pattern of recurrence. For these reasons, a more judicious and selective use of radiation therapy was suggested. Unfortunately, the slow-growing nature of the neoplasm and the low prevalence of the disease make prospective randomized studies evaluating the role of adjuvant RT following

---

Box 1
The most important determinants influencing the development of recurrence in thymomas

Well-recognized

Stage at presentation

Completeness of resection with safe surgical margins

World Health Organization histology

Suggested

Great vessels invasion

Large-size tumor

resection of thymoma highly unlikely to be undertaken. Several studies, however, have been published in the last 15 years, and although a unanimous consensus has not been reached, some general guidelines for adjuvant radiotherapy may be suggested stage by stage:

Stage 1

The current indications at this stage suggest that adjuvant RT is not indicated, because the recurrence rate is close to 0%,[29,30] Stage 1 thymomas usually are resected completely, and histology is usually type A or B1 (**Table 1**).[3–6,23,24,30–32]

Stage 2

At this stage, RT was offered routinely in the past on the basis of the beneficial effects reported in some studies.[23,24,33,34] Some authors, however, demonstrated that RT does not add any advantage for completely resected stage 2 thymoma.[29,30,35–37] The addition of histologic subtyping is a reasonable approach to fine-tuning the decision to perform RT: A type tumors do not require adjuvant RT while it might be indicated for a B2/B3 lesions. **Table 2** II thymoma.[4,6,23,30,31,33–36] Thus, RT should be reserved in case of close proximity of the tumor to the resection margins or extracapsular involvement of the mediastinal fat or presence of adhesions to the pericardium and mediastinal pleura; it should be considered also in case of a more aggressive histology according to the WHO classification.

Stage 3

This stage includes tumors with macroscopic invasion into neighboring organs with (A) or without (B) involvement of the great vessels. Also at this stage, postoperative RT was administered routinely, and it was considered the gold standard.[32,34] The basis for this recommendation, however, is not clear; the recurrence rates and survival at this stage are reported in **Table 3**.[3,4,6,23,30,31,34,35,38] All but two studies,[23,34] however, which suffered from selection biases, were unable to demonstrate the potential impact of adjuvant RT on recurrence and survival. Other authors found a detrimental effect of RT on recurrence[4]; overall, postoperative RT did not decrease the recurrence rate, and there was no survival advantage. It therefore may be concluded that routine RT in resected stage 3 thymomas should not be indicated. As for other stages, completeness of resection and WHO histology should guide the decision to administer RT after surgery. In experienced centers, the most stage 3 thymomas either with or without the administration of induction chemotherapy may be resected completely (about 80% of the cases).[38] RT should be considered only for patients receiving incomplete resection or with suspected involvement of the surgical margins (ie, tumors peeled off the phrenic nerve with a very close resection margin, **Fig. 1**), or with an aggressive histology (type B2/B3) or, as suggested by some authors, in case of previous open biopsy that could contribute to contaminate the surgical wound. It is important to remind that most of the recurrences after

Table 1
Treatment strategy of stage 1 thymomas in different institutions

Author (Year)	Treatment	Number of Patients	Recurrences	Survival
Curran (1988)	Surgery	42	0	67% (5 y)
Quintanilla (1994)	Surgery	52	0	100% (5 y)
Blumberg (1995)	Surgery	25	1	95% (5 y) 86% (10 y)
Pollack (1992)	Surgery + RT	5	1	
Nakahara (1988)	Surgery or surgery + RT	12 38	1 0	
Singhal (2003)	Surgery or surgery + RT	27 3	1	
Kondo (2003)	Mostly surgery	522	4	100% (5 y)
Haniuda (2001)	Surgery	39	0	
Ruffini (1997)	Surgery or surgery + RT	145 7	7 0	

Abbreviation: RT, radiation therapy.

Table 2
Recurrence rates in stage 2 thymomas with and without postoperative radiation therapy among the largest series published over the last 30 years

Author (Year)	With Radiation Therapy (RT)[a]	Without RT[a]	Conclusions	Survival Advantage of RT
Kondo (2003)	4.7	4.1	No benefit	No survival differences
Quintanilla (1994)	28	8	No benefit	
Haniuda (1992)	23	25	No benefit	
Monden (1985)	8	29	RT beneficial	
Curran (1988)	0	42	RT beneficial[b]	No survival difference
Ogawa (2002)	10		RT beneficial	No survival difference
Ruffini (1997)	31	4	RT detrimental	No survival difference
Rena (2007)	12	6	No benefit	
Singhal (2003)	0.5	0	No benefit	

[a] Recurrence rates in percentages.
[b] Statistical analysis not performed because of a single patient in the no-radiation arm.

resection of stage 3 thymomas are within the pleura rather than the mediastinum, and this should suggest a potential role for postoperative chemotherapy.[38]

Stage 4A

Seven percent to 10% of the lesions are at this stage. Primary surgery still is debated, with a resectability rate of about 40%. Limited pleural-based metastases can be resected completely after cisplatin-based combination chemotherapy, and occasional long-term survival has been reported.[39–41] In most cases, however, pleural dissemination with droplet metastases is evident at inspection of the pleural surface, and in these cases,

debulking within a multimodality protocol has been proposed.[41] Controversy still exists, however, because prolonged survival has been observed with chemotherapy and RT alone.[42,43] Other treatment strategies at this stage include immunosuppressive therapy,[44] surgical removal followed by intrapleural hyperthermic chemotherapy,[45] and extrapleural pneumonectomy (EPP).[41,46,47] The rate of complete resection at this stage is not high, and pleural recurrence after resection has been reported to be as high as 40%. Carcinomatosis is the most frequent pattern of recurrence after complete resection; pleural relapse may occur at any time after surgery, although the mean disease-free interval is between 60 and 80 months. Histology of

Table 3
Recurrence rates in stage 3 thymomas with and without postoperative radiation therapy among the largest series published over the last 30 years

Author (Year)	With Radiation Therapy (RT)[a]	Without RT[a]	Conclusions	Survival Advantage of RT
Kondo (2003)	23	26	No benefit	No survival differences
Quintanilla (1994)	13	13	No benefit	
Haniuda (1992)	30	25	No benefit	
Monden (1985)	24	40	RT beneficial	
Curran (1988)	0	44	RT beneficial[b]	No survival difference
Blumberg (1995)	48	52	No benefit	No survival difference
Ruffini (1997)	64	16	RT detrimental	No survival difference
Mangi (2005)	32	29	No benefit	No survival difference
Singhal (2003)	0.5	0	No benefit	

[a] Recurrence rates in percentages.
[b] Statistical analysis not performed because of a single patient in the no-radiation arm.

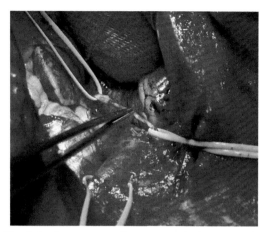

Fig. 1. During surgery for recurrent thymoma the phrenic nerve must be preserved whenever possible to reduce postoperative pulmonary complications.

the pleural implants may be the same as the primary tumor, although sometimes they may be more undifferentiated. In these cases, the most frequent histology is type B3.

THE ROLE OF SURGERY FOR RECURRENT THYMOMA

Only five studies have been published in the international literature during the last 15 years addressing specifically treatment of recurrent thymoma. The small size of the studies, (ranging from 16 to 30 patients), the different patterns of recurrence described (local, pleural and distant), and the relatively long period of time considered (from 1995 to 2005) make comparison difficult (**Tables 4** and **5**).[3–5,8,22,48]

Blumberg and associates in 1995[3] reported on 25 patients who had recurrent thymoma out of 86 resected tumors (29%). Mean time to recurrence was 48 months. Most of their patients had local recurrences (17 patients, 68%). Surgery was performed in 13 patients, with a 5-year survival rate of 45%; however, local recurrence increased to 80% after surgery. The authors concluded that surgery may be indicated, but results are better when treating local recurrence. Ruffini and colleagues in 1996[4] reported on 30 recurrent tumors (11% of the total number of resected patients); the mean time to recurrence was 86 months. In that group of patients, 13 (43%) had pleural recurrence; 11 (36%) had local recurrence; and 6 (20%) had distant metastases. Sixteen patients (53%) underwent surgery, and complete resection was feasible only in 10 cases (62%). Overall, 5-year survival and 10-year survival were 48% and 24% respectively; patients receiving complete resection showed an excellent prognosis (72% 5-year survival). The authors concluded that surgical resection of recurrent

Table 4
Results of surgical treatment of recurrent thymomas among the largest series published in the last 20 years

Author (Year)	Total	Recurrence (%)	Site	Surgery	Complete Resection	Mean Time to Recurrence	Survival (Years)
Haniuda (2001)	126	24 (19%)	22 Pl 6 Loc 5 Dis	15/24	4/15 (27%)	68	47% (5 y) 35% (10 y)
Ruffini (1997)	266	30 (11%)	13 Pl 11 Loc 4 Dis	16/30	10/16 (62%)	86	48% (5 y) 24% (10 y)
Regnard (1997)	285	28 (10%)	15 Pl 8 Loc 5 Dis	28/28	19/28 (68%)	88	51% (5 y) 43% (10 y)
Ciccone (2005)	211	16 (7.5%)	8 Pl 2 Loc 6 Dis	16/16	N.S.	N.S.	64% (5 y) 44% (10 y)
Wright (2005)	179	20 (11%)	16 Pl 2 Loc 2 Dis	N.S.	N.S.	N.S.	N.S.
Blumberg (1995)	86	25 (29%)	1 Pl 17 Loc 7 Dis	13/25	N.S.	48	65% (5 y)

Abbreviations: Pl, pleural recurrence; Loc, local recurrence; Dis, distant recurrence; N.S., not stated in the paper.

Table 5
Conclusions and recommendations about surgery in the treatment of recurrent thymomas among the most representative series over the last 20 years

Author (Year)	Conclusions About Recurrence	Role of Surgery
Haniuda (2001)	Poor prognosis in case of reoperation, although all radically operated cases were alive at 48 months mean follow-up Reoperation should be attempted very selectively only in local recurrence	Rarely recommended
Ruffini (1997)	Surgery recommended in case of recurrence of thymoma Best results in case of local recurrence and total resection of the recurrence	Recommended
Regnard (1996)	Surgery recommended in most recurrent thymomas Recurrence can occur in the thymus left in place at the time of primary surgery, and in the thoracic cavity opened during the first operation Scar recurrence also observed	Recommended
Ciccone (2005)	Surgery recommended Recurrent thymomas occur more frequently in cortical tumors Early recurrence (<40 months) carries a poor prognosis	Recommended
Wright (2005)	Stage, WHO histology, and tumor size (>8 cm) independent predictors of recurrence No need to split Masaoka stage 1 and 2 for recurrence analysis WHO histology may be grouped into four classes: type A (A and AB), early B (B1 and B2), B3, and type C	Not stated
Blumberg (1995)	Surgery recommended in case of local recurrenceLarger tumors associated with a poor prognosis	Recommended

thymoma is appropriate, and an excellent prognosis can be anticipated in case of complete resection of local recurrence.

Similar results were reported in 1997 by Regnard and colleagues[8] on 28 patients out of 288 resected thymomas (10% recurrence rate). The mean time to recurrence was 88 months; pleural recurrence occurred in 53% of the patients, and local recurrence in 28%. Surgery was attempted in all patients. Complete resection was achieved in 19 patients (68%); 5-year survival and 10-year survival were 51% and 47% respectively. It was 64% at 5 years in case of complete resection. On the basis of these findings, the authors strongly recommend surgery in case of recurrence. They also reported that some patients had scar recurrence and observed that most pleural implants occurred when the thoracic cavity was opened during the first operation. In 2001, Haniuda and colleagues[5] reported their experience on 24

patients who had recurrent thymoma out of 126 resected tumors (19%). The mean time to recurrence was 68 months; pleural recurrence was observed in most patients (22 out of 24, 92%). Surgery was attempted in 15 patients, but complete resection was feasible in 4 patients only (27%), with a 5- and 10-year survival rates of 47% and 35% respectively. The authors observed that surgery may not be indicated for all patients who have recurrent thymoma, and they recommended a careful preoperative selection; however, the four patients receiving complete resection were alive 48 months after surgery.

Ciccone and colleagues in 2005[48] reported on 16 patients who had recurrent thymoma out of 211 resected tumors (7.5%). Pleural recurrence was observed in eight cases (50%); all the lesions had cortical differentiation, and in 40% of them, histologic progression was observed. All patients underwent surgery, with a 5-year survival of 64%

in case of complete resection. In that study, a time-to-recurrence below 40 months was associated with poor prognosis.

Surgery for recurrent thymoma (**Box 2**) thus is indicated if complete resection is feasible. The type of surgical approach depends upon the site and side of the recurrence, the associated surgical risks for bone infection, and the surgeon's preference. Pleural recurrences are approached best by means of thoracotomy, although recent reports indicate that sternotomy may be performed; mediastinal recurrence usually is approached by means of median sternotomy. The combination of median sternotomy and anterior thoracotomy may improve exposure of the mediastinum and the ipsilateral hemithorax (**Fig. 2**). A hemi-clamshell, full clamshell, or clamshell extended with a partial sternotomy has been proposed to provide optimal exposure of the mediastinum and the pleural space. Median sternotomy followed immediately by a posterolateral thoracotomy may be an excellent alternative to achieve the best exposure to the mediastinum and the hemithorax.[41,47] In the four major series reporting on surgery for recurrent thymoma, resternotomy was used in 48 cases (five partial sternotomy), and thoracotomy in 44; however, the risk of a re-sternotomy should not be underestimated. In many cases, there are adhesions between sternum and the pericardium or the heart if the pericardium was removed en bloc with the tumor during the first operation (**Fig. 3**); sternal infection increases in diabetic patients or those receiving steroids and other immunosuppressive drugs.

In patients in whom surgery is deemed unfeasible, chemotherapy and radiation therapy should be considered as alternatives.

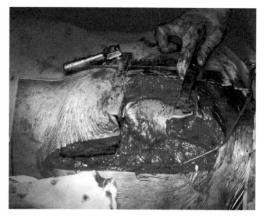

Fig. 2. A combined sternotomy and anterior thoracotomy provides superb exposure to the mediastinum and ipsilateral hemithorax.

Particular attention should be paid to pleural recurrence of thymoma. In fact, it has been demonstrated that a survival advantage can be offered only if complete resection is feasible. Pleural recurrence may occur with large-based single pleural implants, or few metastatic droplets in the costo-diaphragmatic recess or on the diaphragm (**Figs. 4** and **5**); in these cases, complete resection may be performed with limited resection of the diaphragm (**Fig. 6**). In these patients, the role of surgery is indisputable. When patients show pleural carcinosis, however, complete resection is more difficult. Some authors suggested radical pleurectomy and even EPP with resection and replacement of the diaphragm.[49,50] In a recent report, Wright[46] treated two recurrent stage 4A B3 thymomas by an EPP as part of a multimodality treatment protocol with a encouraging outcome; one

Box 2
Prognostic factors in surgically treated recurrent thymomas
Favorable prognostic factors in recurrent thymomas
Surgically amenable recurrence
Local recurrence (confined to mediastinum or lung or limited pleural involvement)
Total resection of the recurrence
Unfavorable prognostic factors in recurrent thymomas
Anatomically unresectable recurrence
Pleural recurrence (multiple droplet metastases)
Incomplete resection of the recurrence

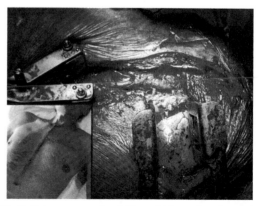

Fig. 3. Extreme care should be paid in performing resternotomy because of the presence of adhesions between the pericardium and the sternum. If difficulties are anticipated on the pleura side, an anterior thoracotomy may be added to gain access to the pleural space.

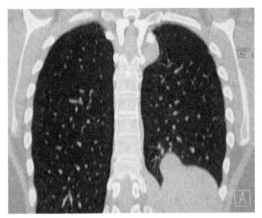

Fig. 4. Coronal CT scan showing recurrence of thymoma as broad-based pleural implants.

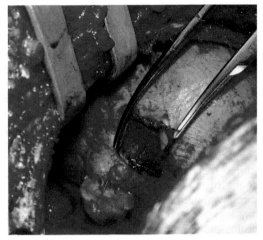

Fig. 6. Pleural recurrence of thymoma: resection of pleural implants on the diaphragm sometimes requires a diaphragmatic resection.

patient died of the disease after 16 years, and the other one had no evidence of disease after 15 years. This operation can be performed through a posterolateral thoracotomy with a second lower intercostal incision to resect and reconstruct the diaphragm (**Fig. 7**); alternatively, the resection can be performed through a median sternotomy as recently proposed for mesothelioma.[51] Strict selection criteria for such an aggressive treatment include young age, excellent cardiopulmonary function, and absence of metastatic disease using positron emission tomography (PET)-CT. Other authors, however, reported a higher mortality with surgery for recurrent thymoma and strongly support alternative treatments such as radiation therapy;[5,52] however, there is no scientific evidence so far that surgery is superior to chemotherapy or radiotherapy in this subset of patients.

Hyperthermic pleural perfusion (HPP) has been described in addition to surgical resection to obtain maximal local control of the disease. Refaely

and colleagues[45] used a Cisplatin perfusate (100 mg/m^2) at an intrapleural temperature between 40°C and 43°C in six patients who had pleural recurrence. They concluded that the technique is feasible and safe, with no mortality and acceptable morbidity; local control was achieved in more than 70% of the patients at 5 years. De Bree and colleagues[53,54] performed debulking and intraoperative hyperthermic intrathoracic perfusion chemotherapy (HITOC) with cisplatin and Adriamicin or doxorubicin with encouraging results.

It therefore seems that, although no evidence-based assumption can be made about optimal treatment of massive pleural recurrence of thymoma, the use of debulking surgery as part of a multidisciplinary approach including low-dose entire

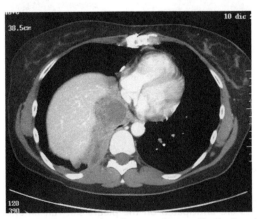

Fig. 5. Axial CT scan showing massive mediastinal and pleural recurrence of thymoma.

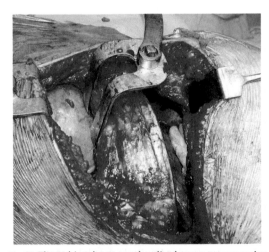

Fig. 7. Pleural implants on the diaphragm may require an additional lower thoracotomy using the same skin incision.

hemithorax radiotherapy (EHRT), HITOC, or HPP is feasible and safe and may be considered as a treatment option. The addition of systemic cisplatin-based chemotherapy or long-term therapy with octreotide analogs has been found to be promising.

THYMIC CARCINOMA

Thymic carcinoma, although traditionally considered together with thymoma, is now an histologically distinct entity; it clearly shows anaplasia, cellular atypia, and increased proliferative activity.[1] This results in a more aggressive clinical behavior with a high recurrence rate. The role of surgery in the treatment of thymic carcinoma still is debated, but it generally is agreed that complete resection is an important therapeutic goal and should be attempted, although it is achieved only in 35% to 50% of the cases.[6,55,56] The role of induction therapy before surgery is unclear, because of the rarity of the disease. The role of surgery in recurrent thymic carcinoma is limited, because recurrence or persistence of thymic carcinoma is almost invariably considered a poor prognostic factor.

THYMIC CARCINOID

Thymic carcinoids are tumors with histologic similarities to their counterparts in the gastrointestinal tract and lung; for this reason, they are considered a separate entity from thymoma. They often are associated with multiple endocrine neoplasia (MEN) syndromes, particularly MEN1. Unlike carcinoids arising elsewhere, thymic carcinoids are aggressive tumors with high recurrence rates and a tendency to give distant metastases.[1] Surgery is the mainstay of therapy. The relapse rate is as high as 60%,[6,57,58] and surgery plays a role also in managing recurrence. Several reports indicate satisfactory long-term survival after resection of the recurrent disease,[58–61] and they suggest that an aggressive approach might be indicated.[62] The role of surgery in recurrent carcinoids is far less clear, however, and the choice of the optimal treatment strategy is based on a personal and individual basis.

SUMMARY

Surgery plays an important role in treating recurrent thymic tumors. This approach may require both induction therapy and oncological consolidation (adjuvant) in case the lesion shows extended invasion of the surrounding organs. Extended resections are justified to achieve complete removal of the recurrence. Recurring thymic carcinoma or carcinoids may be more difficult to treat.

REFERENCES

1. Pearson FG. Thoracic surgery. Philadelphia: Churchill Livingstone; 2002.
2. Maggi G, Casadio C, Cavallo A, et al. Thymoma: results of 241 operated cases. Ann Thorac Surg 1991;51:152–6.
3. Blumberg D, Port JL, Weksler B, et al. Thymoma: a multivariate analysis of factors predicting survival. Ann Thorac Surg 1995;60:908–14.
4. Ruffini E, Mancuso M, Oliaro A, et al. Recurrence of thymoma: analysis of clinicopathologic features, treatment, and outcome. J Thorac Cardiovasc Surg 1997;113:55–63.
5. Haniuda M, Kondo R, Numanami H, et al. Recurrence of thymoma: clinicopathological features, reoperation, and outcome. J Surg Oncol 2001;78:183–8.
6. Kondo K, Monden Y. Therapy for thymic epithelial tumors: a clinical study of 1320 patients from Japan. Ann Thorac Surg 2003;76:878–85.
7. Venuta F, Rendina EA, Longo F, et al. Long-term outcome after multimodality treatment for stage III thymic tumors. Ann Thorac Surg 2003;76:1866–72.
8. Regnard JF, Zinzindohoue F, Magdeleinat P, et al. Results of reresection for recurrent thymomas. Ann Thorac Surg 1997;64:1593–8.
9. Kaiser LR. Thymoma. The use of minimally invasive resection techniques. Chest Surg Clin N Am 1994;4(1):185–94.
10. Bodner J, Wykypiel H, Greiner A, et al. Early experience with robot-assisted surgery for mediastinal masses. Ann Thorac Surg 2004;78(1):259–65.
11. Lucchi M, Basolo F, Mussi A. Surgical treatment of pleural recurrence from thymoma. Eur J Cardiothorac Surg 2008;33:707–11.
12. Okumura M, Otha M, Tateyama H, et al. The World Health Organization histologic classification system reflects the oncologic behaviour of thymoma. A clinical study of 273 patients. Cancer 2002;94:624–32.
13. Kondo K, Yoshizawa K, Tsuyuguchi M, et al. WHO histologic classification is a prognostic indicator in thymoma. Ann Thorac Surg 2004;77:1183–8.
14. Rena O, Papalia E, Maggi G, et al. World Health Organization histologic classification: an independent prognostic factor in resected thymomas. Lung Cancer 2005;50:59–66.
15. Park MS, Chung KY, Kim KD, et al. Prognosis of thymic epithelial tumors according to the new World Health Organization histologic classification. Ann Thorac Surg 2004;78:992–8.
16. Okumura M, Miyoshi S, Takeuchi Y, et al. Results of surgical treatment of thymomas with special reference to the involved organs. J Thorac Cardiovasc Surg 1999;117:605–13.

17. Masaoka A, Monden Y, Nakahara K, et al. Follow-up study of thymomas with special reference to their clinical stages. Cancer 1981;48:2485–92.

18. Masaoka A, Yamakawa Y, Niwa H, et al. Thymectomy and malignancy. Eur J Cardiothorac Surg 1994;8:251–3.

19. Haniuda M, Miyazawa M, Yoshida K, et al. Is postoperative radiotherapy for thymoma effective? Ann Surg 1996;224(2):219–24.

20. Rosai J, Sobin LH. World Health Organization, International Histological Classification of Tumors. Histological typing of tumors of the thymus. 2nd edition. Berlin: Springer-Verlag; 1999.

21. Strobel P, Marx A, Zettl A, et al. Thymoma and thymic carcinoma: an update of the WHO classification 2004. Surg Today 2005;35:805–11.

22. Wright CD, Wain JC, Wong DR, et al. Predictors of recurrence in thymic tumors: importance of invasion, World Health Organization histology and size. J Thorac Cardiovasc Surg 2005;130:1413–21.

23. Curran WJ, Kornstein FJ, Brooks JJ, et al. Invasive thymoma: the role of mediastinal irradiation following complete or incomplete surgical resection. J Clin Oncol 1988;6:1722–77.

24. Pollack A, Komaki R, Cox JD, et al. Thymoma: treatment and prognosis. Int J Radiat Oncol Biol Phys 1992;23:1037–43.

25. Myojin M, Choi NC, Wright CD, et al. Stage III thymoma: pattern of failure after surgery and postoperative radiotherapy and its implication for future study. Int J Radiat Oncol Biol Phys 2000;46:927–33.

26. Kleikamp G, Schnepper U, Korfer R. Coronary artery disease and aortic valve disease as a long-term sequel of mediastinal and thoracic irradiation. J Thorac Cardiovasc Surg 1997;45:27–31.

27. Shulimzon T, Apter S, Weitzen R, et al. Radiation pneumonitis complicating mediastinal radiotherapy postpneumonectomy. Eur Respir J 1996;9:2697–9.

28. Yeoh E, Holloway RH, Russo A, et al. Effects of mediastinal irradiation on esophageal function. Gut 1996;38:166–70.

29. Wright CD. Management of thymomas. Crit Rev Oncol Hematol 2008;65:109–20.

30. Singhal S, Shrager JB, Rosenthal DI, et al. Comparison of stages: thymoma-treated complete resection with or without adjuvant radiation. Ann Thorac Surg 2003;76:1635–42.

31. Quintanilla-Martinez L, Wilkins EW, Choi NC, et al. Thymoma. Histologic subclassification is an independent prognostic factor. Cancer 1994;74:606–17.

32. Nakahara K, Ohno K, Hashimoto J, et al. Thymoma: results with complete resection and adjuvant postoperative irradiation in 141 consecutive patients. J Thorac Cardiovasc Surg 1988;95:1041–7.

33. Ogawa K, Uno T, Toita T, et al. Postoperative radiotherapy for patients with completely resected thymoma. Cancer 2002;94:1405–13.

34. Monden Y, Nakahara K, Iioka S, et al. Recurrence of thymoma: clinicopathological features, therapy, and prognosis. Ann Thorac Surg 1985;39:165–9.

35. Haniuda M, Morimoto M, Nishimura H, et al. Adjuvant radiotherapy after complete resection of thymoma. Ann Thorac Surg 1992;54:311–5.

36. Rena O, Papalia E, Oliaro A, et al. Does adjuvant radiation therapy improve disease-free survival in completely resected Masaoka stage II thymoma? Eur J Cardiothorac Surg 2007;31:109–13.

37. Mangi AA, Wright CD, Allan JS, et al. Adjuvant radiation therapy for stage II thymoma. Ann Thorac Surg 2002;74(4):1033–7.

38. Mangi AA, Wain JC, Donahue DM, et al. Adjuvant radiation of stage III thymoma: is it necessary? Ann Thorac Surg 2005;79(6):1834–9.

39. Kim ES, Putnam JB, Komaki R, et al. Phase II study of a multidisciplinary approach with induction chemotherapy followed by surgical resection, radiation therapy and consolidation chemotherapy for unresectable malignant thymomas: final report. Lung Cancer 2004;44:369–79.

40. Lucchi M, Ambrogi MC, Duranti L, et al. Advanced-stage thymomas and thymic carcinomas: results of multimodality treatments. Ann Thorac Surg 2005;79:1840–4.

41. Huang J, Riely GJ, Rosenzweig KE, et al. Multimodality therapy for locally advanced thymomas: state of the art or investigational therapy? Ann Thorac Surg 2008;85:365–7.

42. Loehrer PJ, Chen M, Kim K, et al. Cisplatin, doxorubicin, and cyclophosphamide in metastatic or recurrent thymoma: an intergroup trial. J Clin Oncol 1997;15:3093–9.

43. Loehrer PJ, Kim KM, Aisner SC, et al. Cisplatin plus doxorubicin plus cyclophosphamide in metastatic or recurrent thymoma: final results of an intergroup trial. J Clin Oncol 1994;12:1164–8.

44. Taguchi T, Suehiro T, Toru K, et al. Pleural dissemination of thymoma showing tumor regression after combined corticosteroid and tacrolimus therapy. Eur J Intern Med 2006;17(8):575–7.

45. Refaely Y, Simansky DA, Paley M, et al. Resection and perfusion thermochemotherapy: a new approach for the treatment of thymic malignancies with pleural spread. Ann Thorac Surg 2001;72:366–70.

46. Wright CD. Pleuropneumonectomy for the treatment of Masaoka stage IVA thymoma. Ann Thorac Surg 2006;82:1234–9.

47. Huang J, Rizk NP, Travis WD, et al. Feasibility of multimodality therapy including extended resections in stage IVA thymoma. J Thorac Cardiovasc Surg 2007;134:1477–84.

48. Ciccone AM, Rendina EA. Treatment of recurrent thymic tumors. Semin Thorac Cardiovasc Surg 2005;17:27–31.

49. Suzuki S, Okada S, Nagamoto N, et al. Pleuropneumonectomy with thymectomy for invasive thymoma

with pleural disseminations. A case report. Nippon Kyobu Geka Gakkai Zasshi 1990;38:1371–4.

50. Shinada J, Yoshimura H, Hirai S, et al. Pleuropneumonectomy with combined resection of diaphragm, superior vena cava, and pericardium for invasive thymoma with pleural dissemination. Kyobu Geka 1991;44:949–52.

51. Martin-Ucar AE, Stewart DJ, West KJ, et al. A median sternotomy approach to right extrapleural pneumonectomy for mesothelioma. Ann Thorac Surg 2005;80:1143–5.

52. Ichinose Y, Ohta M, Yano T, et al. Treatment of invasive thymoma with pleural dissemination. J Surg Oncol 1993;54(3):180–3.

53. De Bree E, Van Ruth S, Baas P, et al. Cytoreductive surgery and intraoperative hyperthermic intrathoracic chemotherapy in patients with malignant mesothelioma or pleural metastases of thymoma. Chest 2002;121(2):480–7.

54. De Bree E, Van Ruth S, Schotborgh CE, et al. Limited cardiotoxicity after extensive thoracic surgery and intraoperative hyperthermic intrathoracic chemotherapy with doxorubicin and cisplatin. Ann Surg Oncol 2007;14(10):3019–26.

55. Hsu CP, Chen CY, Chen CL, et al. Thymic carcinoma. Ten years' experience in twenty patients. J Thorac Cardiovasc Surg 1994;107:615–20.

56. Suster S, Rosai J. Thymic carcinoma. A clinicopathologic study of 60 cases. Cancer 1991;67:1025–32.

57. Moran CA, Suster S. Neuroendocrine carcinomas (carcinoid tumor) of the thymus. Am J Clin Pathol 2000;114:100–10.

58. Fukai I, Masaoka A, Fujii Y, et al. Thymic neuroendocrine tumor (thymic carcinoid): a clinicopathologic study in 15 patients. Ann Thorac Surg 1999;67:208–11.

59. Nakagawa K, Yasumitsu T, Kotake Y, et al. Thymic carcinoid tumor—report of 3 operated cases. Nippon Kyobu Geka Gakkai Zasshi 1992;40:1955–61.

60. Economopoulos GC, Lewis JW Jr, Lee MW, et al. Carcinoid tumours of the thymus. Ann Thorac Surg 1990;50:58–63.

61. Wang DY, Chang DB, Kuo SH, et al. Carcinoid tumors of the thymus. Thorax 1994;49:357–61.

62. Sakuragi T, Rikitake K, Nastuaki M, et al. Complete resection of recurrent thymic carcinoid using cardiopulmonary bypass. Eur J Cardiothorac Surg 2002;21:152–4.

Advances in Radiotherapy for Tumors Involving the Mediastinum

Kevin S. Choe, MD, PhD[a], Joseph K. Salama, MD[a,b,c],*

KEYWORDS

- Radiotherapy • Radiation therapy
- Mediastinum • Innovations

The mediastinum is the central region of the thorax, which contains structures important for the routine functioning of the circulatory, nervous, gastrointestinal, respiratory, and lymphatic systems. Benign and malignant tumors arising from structures within the mediastinum are relatively uncommon, and these include thymomas, thymic carcinomas, thyroid cancer, germ cell tumors, lymphomas, and esophageal tumors. More often, neoplasms involving the mediastinum are caused by the metastatic involvement of mediastinal lymph nodes. As primary and metastatic mediastinal tumors arise among critical organs, their management often requires radiotherapy (RT) delivered neoadjuvantly or adjuvantly to surgical intervention. Recent innovations in radiotherapy allow for improved tumor targeting and more precise radiation dose delivery. This article describes diseases of the mediastinum commonly treated with RT, and how innovations in RT planning and delivery specifically apply to tumors within the mediastinum.

MEDIASTINAL DISEASES REQUIRING RADIATION THERAPY
Thymoma

Thymomas are the most common neoplasms of the anterior mediastinum, representing about 20% to 30% of anterior mediastinal masses.[1,2]

The growth of thymomas is usually characterized as indolent, and the cells often lack cytologic features of malignancy. Typically, they invade locally into surrounding tissues, but they rarely can metastasize within the thorax or to extrathoracic sites hematogenously or lymphogenously.[3]

Complete surgical resection is the cornerstone of management, as it is not only therapeutic but also provides prognostic information. The presence of invasion is an important adverse prognostic factor, that is associated with a high propensity for disease recurrence.[4] Other prognostic factors include tumor size, histologic type, and stage. For noninvasive encapsulated thymomas (stage 1), local control is nearly 100% with complete resection alone. For thymomas with capsular invasion (stage 2) or invasion into surrounding structures (stage 3), however, postoperative RT is indicated even after complete resection. RT is effective in reducing mediastinal relapse following surgery in stage 2 and 3 diseases, with the 5-year actuarial mediastinal relapse rate reduced from 53% to 0% in one series and from 28% to 5% in a pooled analysis.[4] Adjuvant RT is important, as salvage rate following recurrence is poor, with up to 63% of relapsing patients dying of progressive disease.[4]

Definitive RT is indicated for patients who have advanced unresectable disease or for those who are poor surgical candidates. Arakawa and

[a] Department of Radiation and Cellular Oncology, University of Chicago, 5758 South Maryland Avenue, MC 9006, Chicago, IL 60637, USA
[b] Cancer Research Center, University of Chicago, Chicago, IL, USA
[c] Ludwig Center for Metastases Research, University of Chicago, Chicago, IL, USA
* Corresponding author. Department of Radiation and Cellular Oncology, University of Chicago, 5758 South Maryland Avenue, MC 9006, Chicago, IL 60637.
E-mail address: jsalama@radonc.uchicago.edu (J.K. Salama).

Thorac Surg Clin 19 (2009) 133–141
doi:10.1016/j.thorsurg.2008.09.010
1547-4127/08/$ – see front matter © 2009 Elsevier Inc. All rights reserved.

colleagues[5] reported the outcome of 12 such patients treated with primary RT. They found that seven were alive at 5 years. Another group reported a 5-year survival rate of 87.5% in eight patients who had stage 4 disease, treated with definitive RT.[6] Combined chemoradiotherapy for advanced disease has demonstrated promising results, with an encouraging 80% complete resection rate and 5-year survival rate of 69%.[7]

The target volume for adjuvant RT should include the entire thymus or tumor bed and any involved organs. According to standard guidelines, a clinical target volume (CTV) and planning target volume (PTV) should be defined. The preoperative CT and fluorodeoxyglucose positron emission tomography (FDG-PET) images, if available, should be used to accurately delineate the tumor bed. Metallic clips placed at the margins of the resection cavity by surgeons also may be very useful. For PTV definition, institutional variation for set-up uncertainty and organ motion should be considered. For patients treated postoperatively, 45 to 50 Gy routinely is delivered in 1.8 to 2.0 Gy daily fractions. For involved margins or gross residual disease, higher doses of up to 60 to 65 Gy may be appropriate, although no radiation dose response has been reported.

Lymphoma

Lymphoma is a relatively common mediastinal tumor, which constitutes about 20% of adult mediastinal tumors and up to 50% of childhood mediastinal malignancies.[8] Although lymphomas are broadly classified into two major groups, Hodgkin's disease (HD) and non-Hodgkin's lymphoma (NHL), the myriad of diseases classified as lymphomas vary widely in presentation, disease characteristics, and prognosis. One characteristic of lymphomas is that they generally respond readily to modest doses of RT. The treatment approach for HD and NHL is continually evolving, with involved field RT (IFRT) as an important component of therapy.

The treatment of HD is a success story of modern oncology, curing most patients. The current treatment paradigms focus on regimens that minimize toxicity without compromising cure rates. A standard approach entails systemic chemotherapy, with 20 to 40 Gy IFRT, based on histology and bulk of disease. IFRT for mediastinal HD typically includes the superior–inferior extent of mediastinal disease before chemotherapy, while allowing for treatment of the postchemotherapy volumes in mediolateral hilar nodes and disease abutting the lung (pushing margins). The standard involved field for mediastinal HD includes the

mediastinum, bilateral supraclavicular nodes, and bilateral hila. In addition to its role in stage I and II diseases, IFRT may be beneficial even in stage III and IV diseases, for those who achieve only partial response to chemotherapy.[9] Currently, the use of RT based on treatment response assessed by FDG-PET is being investigated, and indications for RT may evolve further.

With excellent cure rates, survivors of HD are at risk for long-term complications secondary to mediastinal irradiation, including secondary malignancies (primarily breast cancer in young women) and cardiovascular and pulmonary injuries. With reduction in doses and field size, the risks for these complications should decrease. Nevertheless, mediastinal irradiation in young patients should be done judiciously, and such patients should be monitored closely with regular physical examinations and mammograms.

Unlike HD, NHL often presents as systemic disease, and its mode of spread is less predictable, with noncontiguous lymph node involvement. Management of NHL is steered by histology and disease extent. Diffuse large B-cell lymphoma (DLBCL) is the most common type of mediastinal NHL. Primary mediastinal B-cell lymphoma (PMBCL) is a subtype of DLBCL that is thought to arise from thymic medullary B-cells, with a propensity to affect younger adults.[10–12] Although most patients who have advanced-stage aggressive lymphoma are treated with combination chemotherapy only, IFRT following systemic chemotherapy is standard therapy for patients who have stage I and II DLBCL.[13]

Non-Small Cell Lung Cancer

Non-small cell lung cancers (NSCLCs) often present with nodal metastases in the mediastinum (stage 3), which correlates with a poor prognosis.[14] For patients who have mediastinal lymph node involvement, platinum-based chemotherapy given in conjunction with RT has been shown to increase survival.[15,16] Although concurrent chemotherapy with RT is more efficacious,[17–19] for the frail or elderly, sequential chemoradiotherapy can be used.[15] For operable stage III patients, the sterilization of mediastinal lymph node micrometastases with neoadjuvant chemoradiotherapy has been shown to result in improved progression-free survival.[20,21] For inoperable patients, dose escalation beyond 60 Gy to only the involved regions is being investigated, as cooperative group studies have demonstrated promising survival rates.[22]

The role of postoperative RT (PORT) following surgical resection for NSCLC patients is controversial, but recent data are elucidating its role. A meta-analysis, which compared surgery versus surgery and PORT, showed a clear detriment to survival in stage I and II patients and a nonsignificant benefit in stage III, N_2 patients.[23,24] Although this study often serves as the basis for treatment recommendations,[25] it included trials from as early as 1966, and the conclusion may reflect outdated staging evaluation and treatment. Indeed many patients were treated with cobalt machines, single RT portals, and a large fraction size. With modern technologies, there is convincing evidence that PORT improves the survival in patients who have N_2 disease. A review of 7465 patients in the Surveillance Epidemiology and End Result (SEER) database revealed a significant survival benefit of PORT in patients who had N_2 disease (hazard ratio = 0.855).[26] Furthermore, the Adjuvant Navelbine International Trialist Association (ANITA) trial showed that patients with pathologic N_2 disease had an improvement in 5-year overall survival, from 34% to 47%, with adjuvant RT.[27,28] A dose of 50 Gy typically is delivered for PORT. Although no benefit has been shown for concurrent postoperative chemoradiotherapy versus radiotherapy,[29] high median survival rates of 56 months have been seen in patients treated prospectively in the cooperative group setting.[30]

Small Cell Lung Cancer

Small cell lung cancer (SCLC) is an aggressive form of lung cancer with rapid growth, and it commonly metastasizes to mediastinal lymph nodes and distant organs. For the one third of patients who have limited-stage disease, the addition of thoracic RT has been shown to provide a 5% absolute survival benefit at 3 years.[31,32] To eradicate lymph node micrometastases, the mediastinum, hilum, and primary tumor mass routinely are treated together. In the setting of concurrent cisplatin and etoposide, twice-daily RT to a dose of 45 Gy is more effective than once-daily RT to 45 Gy.[33] Currently, the effectiveness of daily RT to 70 Gy is being compared with twice daily RT, delivered either twice daily to 45 Gy (1.5 Gy twice daily) or delayed concomitant boost to 61.2 Gy (1.8 Gy twice daily in the last 9 days).

CHALLENGES TO RADIOTHERAPY FOR MEDIASTINAL TUMORS

As illustrated, RT long has played a role in managing mediastinal tumors. The delivery of small daily fractions (1.8 to 2 Gy) of ionizing radiation (generated from the bombardment of a tungsten target by electrons) or gamma rays (generated from the decay of radioactive sources) classically induces lethal double-stranded DNA breaks. The daily administration of fractionated RT allows for repair to surrounding normal tissues, while the accumulation of dose within volumes harboring microscopic disease ($\sim$50 Gy), regions of positive margins ($\sim$60 to 66 Gy), and volumes of gross disease ($\sim$66 to 74 Gy) can eradicate tumor.

The ability of RT to sterilize the mediastinal nodal metastases before surgery improves mediastinal control and survival following surgical resection, and its use as a definitive treatment for medically inoperable and technically unresectable patients is established. Classically, RT was delivered to the mediastinum by means of anterior–posterior and posterior–anterior opposed beam arrangements, with the radiation dose prescribed to one central point or a few specific points within the treatment field in the midplane of the patient. RT field borders were standardized to osseous anatomic landmarks, and modified based on the location of surgical clips. These conventional radiotherapy methods encompassed most mediastinal structures. Typical mediastinal radiotherapy fields included the entire mediastinum, extending from the thoracic inlet superiorly to 5 cm below the carina, and extending laterally 2 cm from the vertebral bodies. Often, bilateral supraclavicular fossae were included. Unfortunately, classical radiotherapy planning and delivery techniques often exposed large volumes of the heart, esophagus, and uninvolved lung to radiation. The resulting potential for severe radiation-induced toxicities, including pericarditis, pericardial effusion, accelerated atherosclerosis, pneumonitis, pulmonary fibrosis, and esophageal stricture limited the utility of RT.

Recent innovations have improved the therapeutic ratio of RT delivered to the mediastinum. Advances in RT for mediastinal malignancies can be grouped into three main categories: improvements in radiotherapy planning, the integration of new radiation modalities, and more precise delivery of radiation.

Improvements in Radiotherapy Planning

Improvements in mediastinal RT originate with improved precision in RT planning. Precise delivery of radiation to targets with sharp dose gradients between tumors and surrounding normal tissues is only possible when patients are positioned precisely, comfortably, and reproducibly for each fraction of radiation. This is achieved with customized immobilization devices. Typically, when targeting the mediastinum with radiation, patients are positioned supine with their arms placed above their head. This position maximizes the number of beam angles that can be used, without treating unnecessarily through the arms. Alternatively, a single arm above the head or arms placed akimbo also can be used. Various materials have been developed to maintain patient positioning, including custom foam casts, vacuum molds, and thermoplastic materials. For patients who require even more precise positioning (eg, for radiosurgery), frames with fiducials are used.

The routine incorporation of CT scans into RT planning has allowed for improved targeting of tumors and avoidance of normal tissues. Dedicated multislice CT simulators for RT are used routinely in practice, and they have shortened image acquisition time and reduced artifacts from respiratory movements.[34,35] Respiratory motion of pulmonary and mediastinal structures can be compensated for by using respiratory control methods, such as abdominal compression and active breathing control. Methods that account for respiratory motion (respiratory gating) or methods that track motion (tracking of implanted fiducials) also are used. FDG-PET and magnetic resonance imaging (MRI) scans can be fused readily to the planning CT to aid tumor delineation. This is especially helpful when planning RT for tumors that have caused downstream atelectasis.

Conformal Radiotherapy

Rather than relying on standardized osseous landmarks to define RT fields, three- dimensional RT planning is based on tumor and normal organ volumes outlined on individual CT slices. To account for patient set-up uncertainty and organ motion, tumor volumes are expanded into a planning target volume (PTV). To minimize the chance of radiation-induced toxicity and maximize the therapeutic ratio, PTV and organs at risk are considered to determine the optimal beam angles and field apertures. The goal of conformal RT is to maximize target coverage, without exceeding the radiation tolerance of nearby normal organs.

Based on the volume of normal organs exposed to specific doses of radiation, the risk of RT-induced toxicity can be predicted. For patients receiving mediastinal RT, doses to the spinal cord, lungs, heart, and esophagus are factors that limit the RT dose that can be delivered safely. Although RT-induced transverse myelitis is the most feared long-term complication, the incidence of this complication is extremely low. When the maximum thoracic RT dose is limited to less than 50 Gy, the incidence of transverse myelitis is less than 1%. More common is pulmonary toxicity, usually in the form of radiation pneumonitis. Acute radiation pneumonitis is characterized by the gradual onset

of a cough, usually not productive, often associated with dyspnea and fever. Analyses of large groups of patients planned with three-dimensional conformal RT (3D-CRT) have elucidated dose–volume metrics associated with pulmonary toxicity. Although many dose–volume metrics have been reported, a mean lung dose (ie, the average dose delivered to the lung) greater than 20 Gy is associated with an increased risk of lung toxicity.[36] Additionally, volumes of tumor-free lung receiving more than 20 Gy greater than 40% are associated with a 36% risk of grade 3–5 pneumonitis.[37] For patients receiving concurrent chemotherapy and radiotherapy, the volume of lung receiving greater than 5 Gy was demonstrated in some series to be the most significant predictor of radiation-induced pulmonary toxicity. Esophagitis is seen more commonly with concurrent chemoradiotherapy, and the risk increases with a maximum dose greater than 58 Gy to the esophagus and with larger volumes of esophagus receiving greater than 60 Gy.[38]

Reducing Uncertainty due to Organ Motion

Tumor motion during respiration represents a major challenge in RT for a large number of tumor sites, but especially for tumors of the thorax and mediastinum. During a respiratory cycle, intrathoracic tumors move and change shape, especially for tumors that are near the diaphragm.[39] The displacement can be as high as 6 to 7 mm in subcarinal and hilar lymph nodes.[40] Respiratory motion complicates the delivery of RT in multiple ways. First, delineation of both normal tissue and tumor volumes may be inaccurate because of organ motion during planning CT acquisition. In addition, the tumor may not reside within the delineated target volume during some phases of the respiratory cycle, which can lead to underdosing of tumors and overdosing of normal tissues. One method to ensure targeting of tumors as they move with respiration is adding a larger margin around the tumor. This consequently leads to irradiation of more normal tissue. The problem with organ motion is amplified as treatments become more conformal, where the precise definition of target and normal tissues is critical.

There are several techniques that have been developed to account for respiratory movement during RT. One widely used method is to measure the amplitude of respiratory movements with fluoroscopy or slow CT acquisition, and generate a target volume with margins that would encompass the tumor at all phases of the respiratory cycle. Although relatively simple, this may lead to irradiation of excessively large volumes of normal tissues. Alternatively, organ motion can be minimized by breath holding, either voluntarily by patients or by obstructing the air flow with a valve.[41,42] Breath–hold usually is performed at deep inspiration, and radiation is delivered only during this period. This technique allows more precise target delineation and lowers the volumes of lung and heart irradiated. A major disadvantage of the breath-holding technique is that it can be used only for select patients, as many patients who have intrathoracic tumors cannot tolerate breath holding for an adequate duration.

A new approach that does not require breath holding is respiratory gating or breathing–synchronized radiation delivery.[43,44] In this technique, patients breathe freely and regularly, with delivery of radiation only during a defined phase or amplitude of the respiratory cycle. This requires a system that tracks the patient's breathing, a planning CT simulator that acquires images only during defined phases of respiration, and a linear accelerator that delivers radiation during the same phases. Because image acquisition and radiation delivery are limited to a portion of the respiratory cycle, simulation and treatment sessions are generally longer.

IMPROVEMENTS IN RADIOTHERAPY DELIVERY
Intensity-Modulated Radiotherapy

Because critical organs surround mediastinal tumors, delivering curative doses of RT can be difficult without increasing the risk of radiation-induced toxicities. With the advent of three-dimensional treatment planning and multiple beam arrangements, RT dose escalation has become possible, while sparing surrounding organs. For stage III$_A$ NSCLCs involving mediastinal lymph nodes, conformal techniques have allowed doses to be escalated to 74 Gy, resulting in impressive 24-month median survival in multiple phase 2 studies.[22,45] One method to increase the dose to tumors while limiting high-dose exposure to normal tissues is intensity-modulated radiotherapy (IMRT). IMRT is a form of 3D-CRT where physician-defined target volumes, beam angles, and normal tissue tolerances are entered into complex computer algorithms that derive the optimal treatment plan by dynamically controlling the intensity of the radiation beam. This allows for a high degree of dose conformity around complex and irregularly shaped tumor volumes.

Compared with 3D-CRT, IMRT improves target coverage and spares normal tissues from high doses of radiation.[46–48] In one study of patients who had stage III–IV or recurrent lung cancer, the use of IMRT led to improved target conformity and reduced the predicted risk for pneumonitis, as the median volumes of lung receiving 10 Gy and 20 Gy (V_{10} and V_{20}) were reduced by 7%

and 10% respectively.[47] Grills and colleagues found that IMRT for lung tumors was associated with higher mean tumor doses and tumor control probabilities compared with optimized 3D-CRT with multiple beam angles, limited 3D-CRT with two to three beams, and traditional RT.[46] These gains primarily were seen in cases with mediastinal nodal involvement. Hopefully, these dosimetric advantages will translate into improved disease control and decreased normal tissue toxicity. Reports of clinical outcome in lung cancer patients treated with IMRT are sparse but encouraging.[49]

Although IMRT can shape the dose distribution more conformally than conventional RT, several technical concerns with IMRT must be considered. Respiratory motion is a greater issue when using IMRT than 3D-CRT. Unlike 3D-CRT, in IMRT, the dose from each beam is not delivered all at once. At each beam angle, the intensity of the beam is modulated by multiple smaller subfields that change with time. With the target moving with respiration, the actual radiation distribution and the total delivered dose may be substantially different than what were planned. On the other hand, because a course of RT is typically over several weeks, the effect of target motion in IMRT may even out through the course of treatment and may not be different than 3D-CRT.[50,51]

Another issue in intrathoracic IMRT is the amount of normal tissue exposed to radiation. IMRT improves coverage of tumor volumes with high radiation doses, but in turn, it increases the areas receiving relatively low, yet potentially damaging doses.[47] The spread of low-dose radiation may be associated with an increased risk for toxicity in radiosensitive organs, such as the lungs, especially in the setting of concurrent chemotherapy. When IMRT was used to treat mesothelioma patients following surgery, 6 of 63 patients died of noncancer-related pulmonary causes (four with pneumonia and two with radiation pneumonitis) within 6 months of the completion of radiotherapy.[52] On multivariate analysis, V_{20} was the only predictive variable for post-IMRT death, with V_{20} greater than 7% resulting in a 42-fold risk of pulmonary-related deaths.

Although IMRT is an attractive new modality for treating intrathoracic malignancy in principle, there are several potential issues that require further investigation. Once long-term outcome data with IMRT become available, its appropriate use will be defined better.

Protons and Carbon Ions

Another approach to improving the therapeutic ratio for patients who have mediastinal tumors is the use of radiation modalities other than photons (x-ray gamma ray). Compared with conventional photon therapy, charged particles, such as protons and carbon ions, offer different physical and biological properties that may be useful in tumors of the mediastinum, particularly in patients who have compromised pulmonary or cardiac functions. Charged particles deposit a great deal of their energy at a given depth, followed by a steep dose fall-off, with almost no dose deposition beyond what is called a Bragg peak (**Fig. 1**). This property can be exploited to deliver higher doses to the target without increasing toxicities to surrounding normal tissues.

Currently, proton therapy is limited to a few institutions, with few reports describing its use for mediastinal and thoracic tumors. Planning studies on lung cancer patients report that proton therapy potentially can reduce the radiation exposure to tumor-free lung, lowering the probability of radiation-induced toxicity. For example, in stage I NSCLC, low-dose exposure, such as V_5 in the contralateral lung, was reduced from 17.6% with 3D-CRT to 0.07% with proton therapy.[53] Furthermore, radiation dose to other critical organs, including spinal cord, heart, and esophagus, also was reduced with proton therapy, compared with photon therapy, either 3D-CRT or IMRT.

Clinical data with modern proton therapy are sparse. Although reports on proton therapy for mediastinal tumors are lacking, preliminary data on high-dose hypofractionated proton therapy in early stage lung cancer show that outcomes are comparable to surgical resection. Hata and colleagues[54] treated patients who had stage I NSCLC with 50 to 60 Gy of proton therapy in 10 fractions. Two-year overall survival and cause-specific survival

rates were 74% and 86%, respectively. There was no treatment-related toxicity greater than grade 3, with medium follow-up of 35 months. In another report, Bush and colleagues[55] conducted a similar study, with similar results. Three-year local control and disease-specific survival were 74% and 72%, respectively. Although these are small studies, survival rates are approaching those obtained with surgery,[14] and it may be a good alternative to surgery for those patients who are not surgical candidates or those who refuse surgery.

Another new radiation modality with charged particles is carbon ion radiotherapy (CIRT). Similar to proton beams, carbon ion beams produce a Bragg peak and abruptly dissipate as energy is lost. Unlike protons, however, whose biologic properties do not differ from photons, carbon ions have relative biological effectiveness that is up to fourfold higher, compared with photons and protons. Because of its favorable physical and biological characteristics, CIRT may improve tumor control without increasing toxicity.

The effectiveness of CIRT has been studied in stage I NSCLC. Miyamoto and colleagues[56] treated 50 patients who had stage I NSCLC with a dose of 72 GyEq, delivered in nine fractions. Thirty-three of these patients were medically inoperable. With minimum follow up of 5 years or until death, local control rate was 94.7%. The overall survival was 50%. No lung toxicity greater than grade 3 was observed. Similar outcomes were reported when doses of 52.8 to 60 GyEq were delivered in four fractions.[57]

Favorable physical and biological properties of charged particles make them an appealing alternative to conventional photon RT, and early clinical data are promising. These technologies are still in their infancy, however, and compared with 3D-CRT and IMRT, planning and delivery of charged particles are still primitive. Further improvement in these areas may translate to a substantial clinical benefit. The main limitation of these new modalities is the prohibitively high cost in construction and operation. Large cyclotrons or synchrotrons are necessary to accelerate heavy particles to a clinically useful speed. There are only five full-scale proton therapy centers in operation in the United States currently. Twelve other proton centers are scheduled open in the near future, however. With more experience and less cost, charged particle radiotherapy may become an important option in treating intrathoracic malignancies.

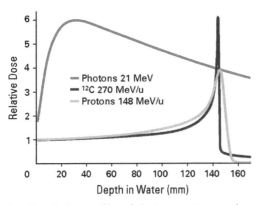

Fig. 1. Depth dose profiles of photons, protons, and carbon ions. *(From* Schulz-Ertner D, Tsujii H. Particle radiation therapy using proton and heavier ion beams. J Clin Oncol 2007;25(8):953–64; with permission. Copyright © 2008 American Society of Clinical Oncology. All rights reserved.)

Stereotactic Body Radiotherapy

The delivery of 1 to 10 high doses (5 to 34 Gy per dose) of radiation to tumors within the body, widely called stereotactic body radiotherapy (SBRT), has gained broad interest recently. This radiotherapy technique is based on the success of stereotactic radiosurgery for central nervous system malignancies, where control of treated tumors approaches 90%. Initially developed at the Karolinska Institute,[58] the delivery of single doses as high as 34 Gy or multiple doses to 60 Gy has resulted in control rates of 80% to 95% for primary and metastatic intrathoracic malignancies.[59] Although control rates are approaching those achieved with surgery, caution must be used when applying this technique to tumors in the mediastinum. Compared with conventionally dosed radiotherapy, SBRT is an ablative therapy, and treatment of tumors within 2 cm of the proximal bronchial tree with high doses (20 to 22 Gy per fraction for three fractions), carries a high risk of grade 3–5 toxicity at 46%.[60] This treatment should be used only for small volumes of gross disease, and it is not intended for treating presumed micrometastatic spread. Unfortunately, normal tissue dose tolerances and optimal dose delivery schedules are unknown with this technique. Widespread application to tumors within the mediastinum should proceed with caution.

SUMMARY

RT is an integral component of treatment in many tumors of the mediastinum. In recent years, there have been advances in RT planning and delivery, which have allowed more effective radiation delivery while sparing normal tissues. New technologies and radiation modalities may help achieve disease control more safely and effectively.

REFERENCES

1. Azarow KS, Pearl RH, Zurcher R, et al. Primary mediastinal masses. A comparison of adult and pediatric populations. J Thorac Cardiovasc Surg 1993; 106(1):67–72.
2. Davis RD Jr, Oldham HN Jr, Sabiston DC Jr. Primary cysts and neoplasms of the mediastinum: recent changes in clinical presentation, methods of diagnosis, management, and results. Ann Thorac Surg 1987;44(3):229–37.
3. Lewis JE, Wick MR, Scheithauer BW, et al. Thymoma. A clinicopathologic review. Cancer 1987;60(11): 2727–43.
4. Curran WJ Jr, Kornstein MJ, Brooks JJ, et al. Invasive thymoma: the role of mediastinal irradiation following complete or incomplete surgical resection. J Clin Oncol. 1988;6(11):1722–7.
5. Arakawa A, Yasunaga T, Saitoh Y, et al. Radiation therapy of invasive thymoma. Int J Radiat Oncol Biol Phys 1990;18(3):529–34.
6. Ichinose Y, Ohta M, Yano T, et al. Treatment of invasive thymoma with pleural dissemination. J Surg Oncol 1993;54(3):180–3.
7. Wright CD, Choi NC, Wain JC, et al. Induction chemoradiotherapy followed by resection for locally advanced Masaoka stage III and IVA thymic tumors. Ann Thorac Surg 2008;85(2):385–9.
8. Priola AM, Priola SM, Cardinale L, et al. The anterior mediastinum: diseases. Radiol Med (Torino) 2006; 111(3):312–42.
9. Aleman BM, Raemaekers JM, Tirelli U, et al. Involved-field radiotherapy for advanced Hodgkin's lymphoma. N Engl J Med 2003;348(24):2396–406.
10. Addis BJ, Isaacson PG. Large cell lymphoma of the mediastinum: a B-cell tumour of probable thymic origin. Histopathology 1986;10(4):379–90.
11. Trump DL, Mann RB. Diffuse large cell and undifferentiated lymphomas with prominent mediastinal involvement. Cancer 1982;50(2):277–82.
12. Waldron JA Jr, Dohring EJ, Farber LR. Primary large cell lymphomas of the mediastinum: an analysis of 20 cases. Semin Diagn Pathol 1985;2(4):281–95.
13. Miller TP, Dahlberg S, Cassady JR, et al. Chemotherapy alone compared with chemotherapy plus radiotherapy for localized intermediate- and high-grade non-Hodgkin's lymphoma. N Engl J Med 1998; 339(1):21–6.
14. Mountain CF. Revisions in the international system for staging lung cancer. Chest 1997;111(6):1710–7.
15. Dillman RO, Seagren SL, Propert KJ, et al. A randomized trial of induction chemotherapy plus high-dose radiation versus radiation alone in stage III nonsmall cell lung cancer. N Engl J Med 1990; 323(14):940–5.
16. Sause W, Kolesar P, Taylor SI, et al. Final results of phase III trial in regionally advanced unresectable nonsmall cell lung cancer: Radiation Therapy Oncology Group, Eastern Cooperative Oncology Group, and Southwest Oncology Group. Chest 2000; 117(2):358–64.
17. Curran W, Scott CB, Langer CJ, et al. Long-term benefit is observed in a phase III comparison of sequential vs. concurrent chemoradiation for patients with unresected stage III NSCLC: RTOG 9410. Proceedings of American Society of Clinical Oncology 2003;22:621 [abstract].
18. Furuse K, Fukuoka M, Kawahara M, et al. Phase III study of concurrent versus sequential thoracic radiotherapy in combination with mitomycin, vindesine, and cisplatin in unresectable stage III nonsmall cell lung cancer. J Clin Oncol. 1999; 17(9):2692–9.
19. Zatloukal PV, Petruzelka L, Zemanova M, et al. Concurrent versus sequential chemoradiotherapy with

Choe & Salama

vinorelbine plus cisplatin in locally advanced non-small cell lung cancer. A randomized phase II study. Proceedings of American Society of Clinical Oncology 2002;21:290A [Abstract].

20. Albain KS, Swann RS, Rusch VR, et al. Phase III study of concurrent chemotherapy and radiotherapy (CT/RT) vs CT/RT followed by surgical resection for stage IIIA (pN2) nonsmall cell lung cancer (NSCLC): outcomes update of North American Intergroup 0139 (RTOG 9309). J Clin Oncol 2005;23(16S):7014.

21. Shaikh AY, Haraf DJ, Salama JK, et al. Chemotherapy and high-dose radiotherapy followed by resection for locally advanced nonsmall cell lung cancers. Am J Clin Oncol 2007;30(3):258–63.

22. Socinski MA, Blackstock AW, Bogart JA, et al. Randomized phase II trial of induction chemotherapy followed by concurrent chemotherapy and dose-escalated thoracic conformal radiotherapy (74 Gy) in stage III nonsmall cell lung cancer: CALGB 30105. J Clin Oncol 2008;26(15):2457–63.

23. PORT Meta-analysis Trialists Group. Postoperative radiotherapy in nonsmall cell lung cancer: systematic review and meta-analysis of individual patient data from nine randomised controlled trials. Lancet 1998;352(9124):257–63.

24. Burdett S, Stewart L. Postoperative radiotherapy in nonsmall cell lung cancer: update of an individual patient data meta-analysis. Lung Cancer. 2005; 47(1):81–3.

25. Bekelman JE, Rosenzweig KE, Bach PB, et al. Trends in the use of postoperative radiotherapy for resected nonsmall cell lung cancer. Int J Radiat Oncol Biol Phys 2006;66(2):492–9.

26. Lally BE, Zelterman D, Colasanto JM, et al. Postoperative radiotherapy for stage II or III nonsmall cell lung cancer using the surveillance, epidemiology, and end results database. J Clin Oncol 2006; 24(19):2998–3006.

27. Douillard JY, Rosell R, De Lena M, et al. Adjuvant vinorelbine plus cisplatin versus observation in patients with completely resected stage IB-IIIA non-small-cell lung cancer (Adjuvant Navelbine International Trialist Association [ANITA]): a randomised controlled trial. Lancet Oncol 2006;7(9): 719–27.

28. Douillard JY, Rosell R, De Lena M, et al. Impact of postoperative radiation therapy on survival in patients with complete resection and stage I, II, or IIIA nonsmall cell lung cancer treated with adjuvant chemotherapy: The Adjuvant Navelbine International Trialist Association (ANITA) randomized trial. Int J Radiat Oncol Biol Phys 2008;72(3):695–701.

29. Keller SM, Adak S, Wagner H, et al. A randomized trial of postoperative adjuvant therapy in patients with completely resected stage II or IIIA non-small-cell lung cancer. Eastern Cooperative Oncology Group. N Engl J Med 2000;343(17):1217–22.

30. Bradley JD, Paulus R, Graham MV, et al. Phase II trial of postoperative adjuvant paclitaxel/carboplatin and thoracic radiotherapy in resected stage II and IIIA nonsmall cell lung cancer: promising long-term results of the Radiation Therapy Oncology Group–RTOG 9705. J Clin Oncol 2005;23(15):3480–7.

31. Pignon JP, Arriagada R, Ihde DC, et al. A meta-analysis of thoracic radiotherapy for small-cell lung cancer. N Engl J Med 1992;327(23):1618–24.

32. Warde P, Payne D. Does thoracic irradiation improve survival and local control in limited-stage small cell carcinoma of the lung? A meta-analysis. J Clin Oncol 1992;10(6):890–5.

33. Turrisi AT 3rd, Kim K, Blum R, et al. Twice-daily compared with once-daily thoracic radiotherapy in limited small-cell lung cancer treated concurrently with cisplatin and etoposide. N Engl J Med 1999; 340(4):265–71.

34. Kalender WA, Polacin A. Physical performance characteristics of spiral CT scanning. Med Phys 1991; 18(5):910–5.

35. Klingenbeck-Regn K, Schaller S, Flohr T, et al. Subsecond multislice computed tomography: basics and applications. Eur J Radiol 1999;31(2):110–24.

36. Seppenwoolde Y, Lebesque JV, de Jaeger K, et al. Comparing different NTCP models that predict the incidence of radiation pneumonitis. Normal tissue complication probability. Int J Radiat Oncol Biol Phys 2003;55(3):724–35.

37. Graham MV, Purdy JA, Emami B, et al. Clinical dose–volume histogram analysis for pneumonitis after 3D treatment for nonsmall cell lung cancer (NSCLC). Int J Radiat Oncol Biol Phys 1999;45(2): 323–9.

38. Bradley J, Movsas B. Radiation esophagitis: predictive factors and preventive strategies. Semin Radiat Oncol 2004;14(4):280–6.

39. Langen KM, Jones DT. Organ motion and its management. Int J Radiat Oncol Biol Phys 2001;50(1): 265–78.

40. Sher DJ, Wolfgang JA, Niemierko A, et al. Quantification of mediastinal and hilar lymph node movement using four-dimensional computed tomography scan: implications for radiation treatment planning. Int J Radiat Oncol Biol Phys 2007;69(5):1402–8.

41. Hanley J, Debois MM, Mah D, et al. Deep inspiration breath-hold technique for lung tumors: the potential value of target immobilization and reduced lung density in dose escalation. Int J Radiat Oncol Biol Phys 1999;45(3):603–11.

42. Wong JW, Sharpe MB, Jaffray DA, et al. The use of active breathing control (ABC) to reduce margin for breathing motion. Int J Radiat Oncol Biol Phys 1999;44(4):911–9.

43. Giraud P, Yorke E, Ford EC, et al. Reduction of organ motion in lung tumors with respiratory gating. Lung Cancer 2006;51(1):41–51.

44. Yorke E, Rosenzweig KE, Wagman R, et al. Interfractional anatomic variation in patients treated with respiration-gated radiotherapy. J Appl Clin Med Phys 2005;6(2):19–32 Spring.

45. Socinski MA, Rosenman JG, Halle J, et al. Dose-escalating conformal thoracic radiation therapy with induction and concurrent carboplatin/paclitaxel in unresectable stage IIIA/B nonsmall cell lung carcinoma: a modified phase I/II trial. Cancer 2001;92(5): 1213–23.

46. Grills IS, Yan D, Martinez AA, et al. Potential for reduced toxicity and dose escalation in the treatment of inoperable nonsmall cell lung cancer: a comparison of intensity-modulated radiation therapy (IMRT), 3D conformal radiation, and elective nodal irradiation. Int J Radiat Oncol Biol Phys 2003;57(3): 875–90.

47. Murshed H, Liu HH, Liao Z, et al. Dose and volume reduction for normal lung using intensity-modulated radiotherapy for advanced-stage nonsmall cell lung cancer. Int J Radiat Oncol Biol Phys 2004;58(4): 1258–67.

48. Xiao Y, Werner-Wasik M, Michalski D, et al. Comparison of three IMRT inverse planning techniques that allow for partial esophagus sparing in patients receiving thoracic radiation therapy for lung cancer. Med Dosim 2004;29(3):210–6 Fall.

49. Sura S, Gupta V, Yorke E, et al. Intensity-modulated radiation therapy (IMRT) for inoperable nonsmall cell lung cancer: the Memorial Sloan-Kettering Cancer Center (MSKCC) experience. Radiother Oncol 2008;87(1):17–23.

50. Bortfeld T, Jokivarsi K, Goitein M, et al. Effects of intrafraction motion on IMRT dose delivery: statistical analysis and simulation. Phys Med Biol 2002; 47(13):2203–20.

51. Chui CS, Yorke E, Hong L. The effects of intrafraction organ motion on the delivery of intensity-modulated field with a multileaf collimator. Med Phys 2003; 30(7):1736–46.

52. Rice DC, Smythe WR, Liao Z, et al. Dose-dependent pulmonary toxicity after postoperative intensity-modulated radiotherapy for malignant pleural mesothelioma. Int J Radiat Oncol Biol Phys 2007;69(2):350–7.

53. Chang JY, Zhang X, Wang X, et al. Significant reduction of normal tissue dose by proton radiotherapy compared with three-dimensional conformal or intensity-modulated radiation therapy in stage I or stage III nonsmall cell lung cancer. Int J Radiat Oncol Biol Phys 2006;65(4):1087–96.

54. Hata M, Tokuuye K, Kagei K, et al. Hypofractionated high-dose proton beam therapy for stage I nonsmall cell lung cancer: preliminary results of a phase I/II clinical study. Int J Radiat Oncol Biol Phys 2007; 68(3):786–93.

55. Bush DA, Slater JD, Shin BB, et al. Hypofractionated proton beam radiotherapy for stage I lung cancer. Chest 2004;126(4):1198–203.

56. Miyamoto T, Baba M, Yamamoto N, et al. Curative treatment of stage I nonsmall cell lung cancer with carbon ion beams using a hypofractionated regimen. Int J Radiat Oncol Biol Phys 2007;67(3):750–8.

57. Miyamoto T, Baba M, Sugane T, et al. Carbon ion radiotherapy for stage I nonsmall cell lung cancer using a regimen of four fractions during 1 week. J Thorac Oncol 2007;2(10):916–26.

58. Blomgren H, Lax I, Naslund I, et al. Stereotactic high dose-fraction radiation therapy of extracranial tumors using an accelerator. Clinical experience of the first thirty-one patients. Acta Oncol 1995;34(6): 861–70.

59. Timmerman RD, Park C, Kavanagh BD. The North American experience with stereotactic body radiation therapy in nonsmall cell lung cancer. J Thorac Oncol. 2007;2(7 Suppl 3):S101–12.

60. Timmerman R, McGarry R, Yiannoutsos C, et al. Excessive toxicity when treating central tumors in a phase II study of stereotactic body radiation therapy for medically inoperable early stage lung cancer. J Clin Oncol 2006;24(30):4833–9.

Index

Note: Page numbers of article titles are in **boldface** type.

Thorac Surg Clin 19 (2009) 143–147
doi:10.1016/S1547-4127(08)00113-8
1547-4127/08/$ – see front matter © 2009 Elsevier Inc. All rights reserved.

Moving?

Make sure your subscription moves with you!

To notify us of your new address, find your **Clinics Account Number** (located on your mailing label above your name), and contact customer service at:

E-mail: elspcs@elsevier.com

800-654-2452 (subscribers in the U.S. & Canada)
314-453-7041 (subscribers outside of the U.S. & Canada)

Fax number: 314-523-5170

Elsevier Periodicals Customer Service
11830 Westline Industrial Drive
St. Louis, MO 63146

*To ensure uninterrupted delivery of your subscription, please notify us at least 4 weeks in advance of move.